Fight Heart Disease

Disease

with Vitamins and Antioxidants

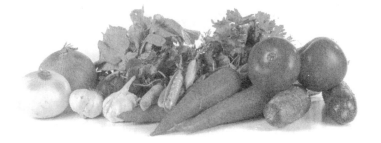

Kedar N. Prasad, Ph.D.

Healing Arts Press

Rochester, Vermont • Toronto, Canada

Healing Arts Press
One Park Street
Rochester, Vermont 05767
www.HealingArtsPress.com

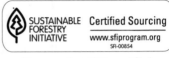

SUSTAINABLE FORESTRY INITIATIVE Certified Sourcing www.sfiprogram.org SFI-00854

Text stock is SFI certified

Healing Arts Press is a division of Inner Traditions International

Note to the reader: This book is intended as an informational guide. The remedies, approaches, and techniques described herein are meant to supplement, and not to be a substitute for, professional medical care or treatment. They should not be used to treat a serious ailment without prior consultation with a qualified health care professional.

Library of Congress Cataloging-in-Publication Data

Prasad, Kedar N.
  Fight heart disease with vitamins and antioxidants / Kedar N. Prasad, Ph.D.
    pages cm
  Includes bibliographical references and index.
  ISBN 978-1-62055-296-4 (paperback) — ISBN 978-1-62055-172-1 (e-book)
  1. Heart—Diseases—Diet therapy. 2. Heart—Diseases—Nutritional aspects. 3. Vitamin therapy. 4. Antioxidants—Therapeutic use. I. Title.
  RC684.D5.P73 2014
  616.1'20654—dc23

                                                            2014015926

Printed and bound in the United States by Lake Book Manufacturing, Inc.
The text stock is SFI certified. The Sustainable Forestry Initiative® program promotes sustainable forest management.

10 9 8 7 6 5 4 3 2 1

Text design and layout by Virginia Scott Bowman
This book was typeset in Garamond Premier Pro and Helvetica Neue with Avant Garde and Helvetica Neue used as display typefaces

To send correspondence to the author of this book, mail a first-class letter to the author c/o Inner Traditions • Bear & Company, One Park Street, Rochester, VT 05767, and we will forward the communication, or contact the author directly at **kprasad@mypmcinside.com.**

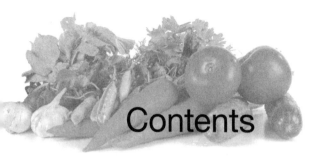

Contents

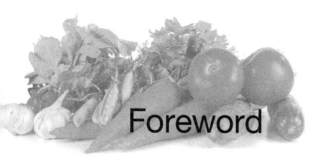

Foreword

Jeffrey L. Boone, M.D.

Medical training encompasses the basics of human nutrition as well as the biochemistry and history of elemental vitaminology and nutrition science. However, as a profession and as a society, we have moved beyond the mere daily allowances required to avoid rickets, scurvy, and the like into a world that demands erudite answers regarding optimal dietary supplementation. As a physician specializing in preventive cardiology, I stood at the center of this controversy amidst patients in search of answers, often skeptical medical colleagues, and a growing body of literature debating the effectiveness of dietary supplementation. Then I met Kedar N. Prasad, Ph.D., a scientist with the brilliance and academic credibility to illuminate the truth with regard to dietary supplements.

I was first attracted to Prasad's work with NASA as a radiation biologist charged with helping to protect military personnel from the dangers of radiation exposure. His groundbreaking work delineated a unique supplement that seemed to protect the subject from the DNA damage and eventual carcinogenesis caused by ionizing radiation. Persuaded by Prasad's detailed research, I began to use his protective formulation of dietary supplements to shield my patients' internal cellular environment from the radiation they received from ultrafast CT scans of the heart. A recent study in Germany showed Prasad's radiation-protection formulation reduced double-strand DNA breakage by 58 percent versus placebo in a study of people before and after diagnostic CT scanning. To this day I continue to use Prasad's formula before CT scans to mitigate the effects of radiation exposure caused by advanced imaging.

As I continued with my work in preventive cardiology, Prasad and his group initiated numerous research trials with disparate groups across the country. I tracked these developments closely, always seeking to remain on the cutting edge of disease prevention. Over the years research emerged that demonstrated a myriad of benefits to Prasad's formulas. Supplement formulations developed around his ideas were shown to enhance immunity, reduce oxidative stress, improve hearing, promote concussion recovery, lessen tinnitus, treat post-traumatic stress disorder, and reduced inflammation! Such widespread benefits can be traced back to the unifying concepts of cellular protection from the basic tenets of Prasad's work—the control of oxidative stress and chronic inflammation. In fact, over the last thirty years it has become increasingly apparent throughout the medical world that most disease and even aging itself can be traced to a core of inflammation and oxidation.

Excited by these widespread applications, I decided to embark upon a research trial in my own field of expertise: the prevention and eradication of heart disease and stroke. Several anecdotal cases of remarkable cholesterol profile improvements were seen in my practice as I expanded my use of Prasad's Heart Formulation beyond radiation protection to daily use in selected patients. These exciting results led Prasad and I to initiate the Boone Heart Institute's MAVRIC Trial (Multivitamin Antioxidant Vitamin Reversal of Intima-Media Thickness of the Carotid Artery). Our study group consisted of seventy robust professional firefighters from South Metro Fire Rescue in Denver, Colorado. They took no medication or other supplements for the duration of the trial. For one year these firefighters took Prasad's Heart Formulation as directed while my medical team tracked their cardiovascular risk factors. As always, the key tenets of the Heart Formulation* revolve around the control of the free radicals causing oxidative stress and chronic inflammation. The Heart Formulation

---

*See www.multimmunity.com for product information.

accomplishes this control through a unique blend of micronutrients that include dietary and endogenous antioxidants coupled with vitamin D, B-vitamins, and minerals (avoiding heavy metals) in a twice-daily dosing schedule. To our amazement, but confirming our hope, Prasad's approach controlled anatomic measurements of the growth of firefighter atherosclerosis, as well as remarkably optimizing the firefighter cholesterol profile (i.e., LDL [bad] cholesterol decreased from 132 mg/DL to 111 mg/DL; HDL [good] cholesterol improved from 42 mg/DL to 51 mg/DL, which constitutes a 30.3% improvement in LDL to HDL ratio). In addition, echocardiographic measurements of heart stiffness (E/A ratio) improved 13 percent. To this day, I recommend Dr. Prasad's formula to many of my patients, often in conjunction with powerful drugs and lifestyle changes.

Read *Fight Heart Disease with Vitamins and Antioxidants* to see how Kedar Prasad has provided us all with a new day of clarity in nutrition science . . . but more importantly, take his formula as I do!

JEFFREY L. BOONE, M.D., is an internationally recognized expert on the effects of mental stress on the heart. He is the founder and director of the Boone Heart Institute in Denver, Colorado. In 2007, he was selected as one of the 160 Top Doctors in America by *Men's Health Magazine* and was listed as one of the seventeen Top Cardiovascular Doctors in America for Men. In addition, he works as a consultant in preventive cardiology for the Denver Broncos and the Colorado Rockies. Dr. Boone is a member of the NFL's Cardiovascular Committee, as well as the founder of the NFL Alumni Association's Cardiovascular Screening Program, an ongoing investigation into the cardiovascular health of former NFL players. As an international lecturer, Dr. Boone has spoken to tens of thousands of health care professionals around the world. His unique clinical approach focuses on aggressive prevention of cardiovascular disease, including the evaluation of the cardiovascular consequences of mental stress, the early clinical use of the latest cardiac imaging techniques, and the advanced detection and treatment of cardiometabolic risk.

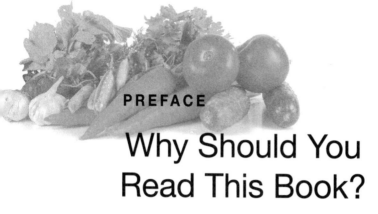

Why Should You Read This Book?

Heart disease remains the number one cause of death in the United States, and death from stroke ranks fourth overall, despite advances in early-disease detection technologies and equipment, and despite current prevention recommendations that involve beneficial changes to one's diet and lifestyle. These startling statistics imply that the prevailing recommendations of the American Heart Association, which involve modifications in diet and lifestyle, are not having the expected and desired results of reducing the prevalence of this disease. If there are no significant changes made to the current preventive recommendations, the projected annual incidence of heart disease in the United States may increase from 981,000 cases in 2010 to 1,234,000 cases in 2040, an increase of approximately 25 percent in thirty years. The number of deaths from this disease is projected to increase from 392,000 in 2010 to 610,000 in 2040, an increase of approximately 56 percent (Odden et al. 2011).

In 2010 the total direct medical cost of heart disease was $273 billion, and the indirect cost (due to lost productivity) was estimated to be roughly $172 billion. By 2030 the projected direct cost will increase to $818 billion and the indirect cost will increase to $276 billion (an increase of approximately 61 percent). These staggering figures make it imperative that we develop an additional strategy to prevent heart disease.

The exact reasons for the failure of the current prevention approaches are unknown. However, it's possible that potential major risk factors for heart disease such as an increased production of free radicals (which leads to increased levels of oxidative stress), chronic inflammation, and the elevated levels of homocysteine that initiate and promote heart disease are not reduced simultaneously by current approaches to prevention. In other words some of these risk factors are targeted by specific approaches that do nothing to address the other risk factors at the same time. This increases morbidity in particular and the overall prevalence of heart disease in general.

Given this, if we were to use antioxidants (that neutralize free radicals and reduce chronic inflammation), and B vitamins (that reduce homocysteine levels), at the same time, we would have an opportunity to reduce these risk factors simultaneously and thereby might reduce the incidence of this disease. Additionally, changes in diet and lifestyle may improve the effectiveness of this strategy.

The current standard care involving medical and surgical procedures has markedly improved treatment outcomes; however, despite these procedures, in any given individual the disease invariably will continue to progress, albeit at a slower rate. This is due to the fact that increased oxidative stress and chronic inflammation continue to exist despite standard care. Thus, supplementation with antioxidants that reduce oxidative stress and chronic inflammation appears to be a very logical choice of treatment protocols for heart disease—to be used in combination with standard care.

Although this is a promising therapeutic model, only a *few* studies with individual antioxidants and omega-3 fatty acids have been performed to test it and *no* studies have been performed to evaluate the efficacy of a micronutrient preparation containing multiple dietary and endogenous antioxidants, B vitamins, vitamin D, omega-3 fatty acids, and certain minerals in combination with standard care.

Antioxidants are usually not recommended by most doctors for the treatment of heart disease. This book clarifies the confusion about the value of antioxidants in this regard. This book also provides scientific data and a rationale for using a preparation of micronutrients containing multiple dietary and endogenous antioxidants, B vitamins, vitamin D, and certain minerals in combination with changes in diet and lifestyle for the prevention and improved management of heart disease. External risk factors (such as obesity, smoking, physical inactivity) and internal risk factors (increased oxidative stress and chronic inflammation) will also be discussed herein, as well as the genetic basis (family history) of heart disease.

Conventional wisdom posits that if heart disease runs in one's family, its onset is inevitable. However, we suggest that familial heart disease can be prevented or delayed by consuming a preparation of multiple micronutrients containing dietary and endogenous antioxidants.

I hope that this book will serve as a guide for consumers when they are selecting an appropriate micronutrient preparation. As well, it is designed to be a guide to specific diet and lifestyle changes that one can make to reduce the risk of heart disease and improve treatment outcomes. Consumers who are taking daily supplements will find the information provided in this book encouraging. Those who are not taking supplements or are uncertain as to their potential benefits may find evidence in these pages that will help them to make a decision about whether or not to take them on a daily basis, in consultation with their doctors.

■ ■ ■

I thank K. Che Prasad, M.S., M.D., for editing this work and for making very valuable suggestions about it.

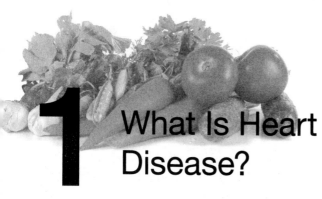

1 What Is Heart Disease?

History, Types, and Cost to Society

As people live longer, the management of chronic diseases, including heart disease, has become increasingly important. Heart disease is a generic term that refers to abnormal conditions of the heart. It may also be referred to as coronary heart disease (CHD), coronary artery disease (CAD), or cardiovascular disease (CVD). It can be caused by changes in heart muscle or in blood vessels that supply blood to the heart or both. Heart disease can lead to stroke, due to a blockage of blood vessels that supply blood to the brain. It can also lead to heart attack, due to a blockage of blood supply to the heart. As we know only too well, strokes and heart attacks may cause death or lead to severe disability.

Today, the prevalence, incidence, and cost of heart disease have been increasing—despite recent advances in its prevention and treatment. The external (outside the body) and internal (inside the body) factors that increase the risk of its development are multiple. Additionally, these risk factors all produce excessive amounts of free radicals and inflammation, which exacerbate conditions of the disease.

This chapter will briefly describe the history of heart disease, as well as the different types of it, and its cost to society. As well, our discussion will provide an overview of other salient facts about it and, in so doing, will provide a basis for the development of an effective strategy to prevent and improve treatment outcomes.

THE HISTORY OF HEART DISEASE

Heart disease, while not a new disease, is one that exists in all mammals. During the course of evolution, mammals developed platelets (fragments of white blood cells), which provided a competitive edge in terms of survival. This is due to the clot-forming property of platelets. Soon after a physical injury, platelets help to form clots at the site of the injury in order to prevent blood loss. Unfortunately, platelets are one of the factors that increase the risk of developing heart disease. We will discuss why this is so in a later portion of this book.

Initially it was presumed that early humans did not suffer from heart disease. This was due in part to the perception that they were physically active and ate meat in conjunction with a diet high in fiber and low in fat. It has also been difficult to find evidence of heart disease among early humans, since neither blood vessels nor heart muscle is capable of being preserved. In centuries past, as today, cremation was a common practice, so finding evidence for heart disease is also difficult for this reason. Also many humans simply did not live long enough for the disease to develop. All of these factors have contributed to the assumption that early humans did not suffer from the effects of this debilitating condition.

The existence of heart disease in early humans remained largely unknown until 2009 when a paper on the topic was presented at a meeting of the American Heart Association (AHA) in Orlando, Florida. This paper reported that computed tomography (CT) scans of ancient Egyptian mummies, some 3,500 years old, revealed evidence of atherosclerosis (hardening of the arteries). The incidence of heart disease in one particular case appears to have been associated with the mature age of the deceased individual. Calcification of the arteries (a hardening of the arteries by calcium deposits) was observed primarily in mummies of people who were older than age forty-five at the time of death. Men and women were equally affected by the disease.

It was reported, as part of the AHA presentation, that a female mummy named Lady Rai displayed evidence of atherosclerosis. This woman had died at the age of thirty or forty in approximately 1530 BCE, which was about three hundred years before Moses lived and about two hundred years before King Tut. It is interesting to note that most of the Egyptian mummies were of people who had enjoyed a high social status. As such they consumed a diet rich in animal fat from such animals as cattle, ducks, and geese. In addition they used salt to preserve their food. It is possible that this high-fat diet, coupled with their excessive salt intake, may have contributed to the development of atherosclerosis (a risk factor for heart disease) among these ancient Egyptians.

In 1513 Leonardo da Vinci, who had no medical training, was among the first to investigate coronary arteries and their functions. In 1628 William Harvey, an English physician, described the circulation of blood, and late in the 1700s, Friedrich Hoffmann, a cardiologist, established the relationship between heart disease and the decreased blood flow found in coronary arteries. In 1706 Raymond de Vieussens, a French anatomy professor, first articulated the structures of the heart's chambers and vessels, and in 1733 Stephen Hales, an English clergyman and scientist, took the progressive step of measuring human blood pressure. In 1912 James B. Herrick, an American physician, offered up the novel suggestion that hardening of the arteries can lead to heart disease.

It is believed that the incidence of heart disease before 1900 was relatively low. It takes a long time to develop heart disease, even among those who are considered to be at high risk. Therefore, the lower incidence of heart disease before 1900 could, in part, be due to the fact that people did not live long enough to develop significant heart disease. There is no doubt that the Industrial Revolution in the West led to marked changes in diet and lifestyle. These changes included the consumption of a high-calorie, low-fiber diet rich in saturated fats and salt, an increase in the smoking of tobacco, and the prevalence of a sedentary lifestyle. These changes in diet and lifestyle caused a marked increase in the incidence of heart disease in the twentieth century.

TYPES OF HEART DISEASE

There are seven types of heart disease that account for almost all heart-related mortality. They include the following:

1. Cardiac arrhythmia (irregular and faster heartbeat)
2. Congenital heart disease (abnormal development of the heart)
3. Heart failure
4. Hypertensive heart disease (systemic and pulmonary)
5. Ischemic heart disease (due to reduced supply of oxygen to the heart)
6. Myocardial disease (damage to heart muscle)
7. Valvular heart disease (damage to the valves of the heart)

Heart disease is complex. Let's examine each of these types of it in greater detail next.

Cardiac Arrhythmia

There are two major types of cardiac arrhythmias: ventricular fibrillation and atrial fibrillation.

Ventricular fibrillation is the most serious of all arrhythmias and results when the heart's ventricles fail to contract and relax in a coordinated manner. This can reduce blood supply to various organs, which can lead to irreversible damage. Ventricular arrhythmias may occur when there is a sudden electric shock to the heart. They may also be due to ischemia (a restriction in blood supply) of the heart muscle. Ventricular fibrillation can occur without atrial fibrillation and, if not treated immediately, invariably causes death.

Atrial fibrillation occurs due to a failure to coordinate contraction and relaxation of the atria and it can take place in the absence of ventricular fibrillation. The mechanism of atrial fibrillation is the same as that of ventricular fibrillation except that it occurs in the atria. Atrial enlargement appears to be a common cause of atrial fibrillation. During atrial fibrillation, the pumping capacity of the ventricles is decreased by only about 20 to 30 percent; therefore, this type of fibrillation does not cause death.

Congenital Heart Disease

This form of heart disease (abnormalities of heart muscle or blood vessels) is generally present at birth. It results from developmental defects that occur during the first three to eight weeks of pregnancy when the major structures of the heart develop. Many fetuses with congenital heart disease die in their mother's womb. However, some survive, although they will typically require fetal heart surgery. In some the disease is not detected until adulthood, when its symptoms begin to present and at which time heart surgery may suddenly be required. The incidence of congenital heart disease is approximately six to eight individuals per one thousand full-term, live births. Genetic factors play a principal role in the development of heart disease. Congenital rubella infection (infection during pregnancy) may also induce it.

Heart Failure

Heart failure occurs when the heart's pumping ability cannot keep up with the demand for blood by various organs of the body. This happens in the pumping chambers of the heart; the ventricles become stiff, and as a result blood cannot properly fill them between heartbeats. It is also possible that the heart muscles become so weak and the ventricles become so dilated that they cannot pump blood efficiently enough to satisfy the needs of all of the organs of the body.

Heart failure may involve the left side, right side, or both sides of the heart. Generally, heart failure begins with the left ventricle. In left-sided heart failure the blood backs up in the lungs, causing shortness of breath.

A viral infection to the heart can cause inflammation of the heart muscles, which is referred to as myocarditis. Myocarditis can lead to left-sided heart failure, which is often associated with right-sided heart failure in that right-sided heart failure typically occurs following left-sided heart failure. When right-sided heart failure occurs, the blood may back up into the abdomen, as well as the legs and feet, causing swelling.

Hypertensive Heart Disease

Systemic hypertension, high blood pressure, or pulmonary hypertension can cause hypertensive heart disease. Systemic hypertension causes hypertrophy (increase in size) of the left ventricle; pulmonary hypertension causes an enlargement of the right ventricle. Increases in the size of the ventricles cause enlargement of the heart. One of the consequences of systemic hypertension is the onset of atrial fibrillation.

Pulmonary hypertensive heart disease may be acute or chronic. Acute pulmonary hypertensive disease can follow a massive pulmonary embolism (the release of a clot or clots into the pulmonary artery). Chronic pulmonary hypertensive disease often causes dilation of the right ventricle. Even mild hypertension (slightly above 140/90 mm Hg), if sufficiently present for a period of time, can cause an enlargement of the left ventricle. Depending upon the severity of the hypertension (high blood pressure), the patients may enjoy a normal life or they may develop progressive ischemic heart disease, leading to heart failure or sudden cardiac death.

Ischemic Heart Disease

Ischemic heart disease results from a poor supply of blood, which reduces oxygen as well as nutrients to the heart, and the inadequate removal of metabolites (waste products) from the heart. The poor blood supply to the heart occurs due to a narrowing of the coronary arteries. The clinical symptoms of ischemic heart disease include the following:

1. Acute myocardial infarction (MI), which can cause the death of heart muscle due to a lack of oxygen
2. Angina, which can cause transient chest pain
3. Chronic ischemic heart disease, which can cause heart failure
4. Sudden death due to a total blockage of the coronary arteries

The symptoms of ischemic heart disease may also occur when plaque ruptures and a blood clot is formed. A large blood clot may partially or completely block the flow of blood through a coronary artery to the heart.

A discussion of the various ways that ischemic heart disease may manifest is what we will look at next.

Acute Myocardial Infarction

Acute myocardial infarction is also commonly referred to as heart attack. It is the most serious form of ischemic heart disease in that it is the leading cause of death in the United States. The annual incidence of MI in the United States is approximately 1.5 million cases, and about half a million people die as a result of acute myocardial infarction per year.

MI causes death of the heart muscle as a result of the disruption of blood supplying the heart. MI can also result from a prolonged and severe reduction in blood pressure, such as may accompany shock and severe hypertension. MI can occur at any age, but its rate of occurrence increases with age and becomes accelerated when atherosclerosis is present.

Approximately 10 percent of MIs occur in individuals under forty years of age. This rate increases to 45 percent for persons under the age of sixty-five, with Caucasians and African Americans equally affected. In general the incidence of MI is higher in men than women and is significantly higher in men when compared to women of reproductive age. The reduced incidence of MI in women of reproductive age may be due to protection provided by the female hormone estrogen. Epidemiologic studies (survey-types of studies) suggest that hormone therapy in postmenopausal women protects against the development of MI, but the same hormone therapy may increase the risk of breast cancer and endometrial cancer. These risks can be markedly reduced by antioxidant supplementation. In laboratory experiments (with animals), estrogen by itself does not cause breast cancer, but it can act as a tumor promoter. The tumor-promoting effect of estrogen can be blocked by antioxidants (Venugopal et al. 2008). Again, this is true in animal experiments; I do not know if this observation is true for humans also.

Creatine kinase is an enzyme present in large amounts in the myocardium of the heart. The activity of this enzyme increases within two to four hours of the onset of MI. It peaks at approximately twenty-four hours and returns to a normal level within seventy-two hours.

The consequences of MI include ventricular dysfunction (failure to pump blood adequately), abnormal arrhythmia, and myocardial (heart muscle) rupture. Deaths that ensue from MI within one year (of an incident of MI) are approximately 30 percent. After that the mortality rate of MI survivors drops to approximately 3 to 4 percent a year.

Angina

Angina is a major symptom of ischemic heart disease in which transient chest pain or discomfort occurs due to a poor blood supply to the heart. There are two major types of angina: stable angina (also called angina pectoris) and unstable angina.

Stable angina is the most common form of angina. It goes away with rest or by taking oral nitroglycerine, a drug that dilates the blood vessels. Like stable angina, unstable angina also causes chest pain (which occurs with increased frequency). The chest pain of unstable angina can occur at rest and for prolonged periods of time. Unstable angina is frequently caused by a disruption of plaque, which can cause thrombosis (blood clots), thereby restricting the blood supply to the heart. This form of angina is a frequent cause of myocardial infarction.

Chronic Ischemic Heart Disease

Chronic ischemic heart disease is observed in patients who have survived the first MI. This form of heart disease can also be associated with a blockage of the coronary artery. Chronic ischemic heart disease is characterized by an enlarged heart, a dilated left ventricle, and moderate to severe stenosis (narrowing) of the coronary arteries.

Sudden Death

Ischemic heart disease can cause sudden cardiac death due to a total blockage of blood supplied to the heart. In the United States, about three hundred thousand to four hundred thousand individuals die of sudden cardiac death every year.

Myocardial Disease

Myocardial disease, also called cardiomyopathy (disease of the heart muscle), results from damage to the myocardium; the heart muscle becomes dilated, as well as increases in size. (About 90 percent of cases of myocardial disease show a dilated form of heart muscle.) Approximately 20 to 30 percent of dilated heart muscle cases have a genetic basis (family history). Myocardial disease associated with an increase in the size of heart muscle is considered a disease of diastolic blood pressure rather than one of systolic blood pressure. About half of these patients (with diastolic blood pressure) have a familial history of myocardial disease. Myocardial disease can cause atrial fibrillation and is the most common cause of sudden death in young athletes.

Valvular Heart Disease

Valvular heart disease of the heart valves can cause stenosis or insufficiency. Stenosis refers to a failure of the heart valve to open completely.

Thus, it interferes with the forward flow of blood. Insufficiency is caused by failure of the valve to close properly, thus allowing blood to flow backward. Valvular defects may occur in one valve or in multiple valves. Impairment in blood flow caused by valvular lesions often produces abnormal heart sounds called murmurs. Valvular lesions may be caused by birth defects or by acquired diseases.

Major valvular lesions include mitral stenosis, mitral insufficiency, and aortic stenosis. Mitral stenosis and aortic stenosis cause about two-thirds of valvular lesions. Valvular lesions can also be a result of calcification, as well as a result of chronic rheumatic heart disease. Acute rheumatic fever caused by bacterial infection (Group A streptococcus pharyngitis) develops in only about 3 percent of patients with this bacterial infection, but it can damage the heart by leading to the development of chronic valvular defects.

PREVALENCE AND INCIDENCE

Heart Disease in the General U.S. Population

Prevalence refers to the estimated number of people who have CHD at a given time, whereas *incidence* refers to the number of new cases of the disease each year. In 2010 the overall prevalence of heart disease in the United States was 6 percent of the population (CDC 2010 Report).

TABLE 1.1. PREVALENCE OF HEART DISEASE IN 2010 IN AGE- AND GENDER-RELATED GROUPS

Age groups (years)	Prevalence (percentage)
60 and over	19.8
45–64	7.1
18–44	1.2
Gender	
Male	7.8
Female	4.6

TABLE 1.2. PREVALENCE OF HEART DISEASE IN 2010 IN RACIAL/ ETHNIC AND GENDER GROUPS

Race/Ethnicity (overall)	Prevalence (percentage)
Caucasian	5.8
African American	6.5
Hispanic	6.1
Asian or Native	3.9
Native American/Native Alaskans	11.6

Levels of education are also related to the prevalence of heart disease. Among individuals who had not obtained a high school diploma, the prevalence of the disease was 9.2 percent. It was 4.6 percent for individuals with a college degree.

In 2004 the annual incidence of heart disease was 1.2 million; this translated to the detection of two new cases per hour in the United States. If there are no significant changes in reducing the impact of risk factors or in improving treatment, the projected annual incidence of heart disease may increase from 981,000 cases in the year 2010 to 1,234,000 cases in the year 2040, an increase of about 25 percent in thirty years.

The prevalence (number of people with heart disease at a given time) of heart disease may increase from 11.7 million in the year 2010 to 17.3 million in the year 2040, an increase of about 47 percent. The number of deaths from heart disease is projected to increase from 392,000 in the year 2010 to 610,000 in the year 2040, an increase of about 56 percent (Odden et al. 2011).

Heart Disease in U.S. Firefighters

A recent examination of duty-specific risks of death from coronary heart disease among on-duty U.S. firefighters revealed that heart disease caused 45 percent of deaths that occurred while the firefighters were on duty (Kales et al. 2007).

In addition it has been determined that the risk of death from heart disease among firefighters is higher than among non-firefighters (Choi 2000). Since 1977 the National Fire Protection Association (NFPA) estimated that between forty and fifty firefighters die on duty every year from cardiac arrest or heart disease.

However, not all of the cardiac events that occurred while firefighters were on duty resulted in death. In 2006 one thousand firefighters suffered an on-duty cardiovascular event that did not result in death (Karter 2007).

It has been reported that heart disease caused 45 percent of the deaths that occurred while they were on duty, compared to 22 percent among police officers, and 11 percent among emergency medical service personnel (Kales et al. 2007).

At present recommendations made by the NFPA and by the National Institute for Occupational Safety and Health (NIOSH) for reducing the risk of heart disease among firefighters are not adequate, because they do not include protection against the excessive amounts of free radicals and inflammation that are produced during the inhalation of smoke and ultrafine air particles; upon heavy physical exertion; and during periods of increased heart rate, heat stress, and intense noise exposure. The increased production of free radicals and toxic agents that accompany chronic inflammation heighten the risk of developing heart disease.

COST TO SOCIETY

As we know heart disease remains the leading cause of death in the United States, and it is estimated that about 17 percent of national health expenditures may be due to this disease. These costs may substantially increase due to increasing numbers of aging people (American Heart Association policy statement, 2011). As stated in the preface to this book, in 2010 the total medical cost of heart disease was $273 billion, and the indirect cost (due to lost productivity) was estimated to be about $172 billion. It is estimated that by 2030 40.5 percent of the population may suffer some form of heart disease. This would increase the direct cost to $818 billion and the indirect cost to $276 billion.

CONCLUDING REMARKS

We tend to think of heart disease as a relatively modern malady. However, the archaeological record reveals that heart disease existed as long ago as 1500 BCE. There are many different ways that heart disease can manifest. The prevalent conditions include cardiac arrhythmia, congenital heart disease, heart failure, hypertensive heart disease, ischemic heart disease, myocardial disease, and valvular heart disease.

The cost to society is enormous. Current expenses add up to hundreds of billions of dollars, and by 2030 the direct cost of heart disease is expected to rise to over 800 billion dollars, with indirect costs estimated to be over 250 billion dollars. It is clear that we need better strategies to combat heart disease, a topic that is the subject of this book.

2 Causes of Heart Disease

The Healthy Human Heart and Risk Factors That Threaten It

The human heart is an amazing organ, and as we continue our discussion, it is essential that we have a basic understanding of its structure and functions as well as its anatomical development. This will allow us to appreciate the complex processes of heart disease better and help us to comprehend how various risk factors may compromise its health.*

ANATOMY

The human heart is a muscular, upside-down, pear-shaped structure located in the chest cavity between the lungs and is made of a special type of muscle cell called myocardium. The heart itself is enclosed in a double-layered membranous sac called the pericardium. The normal weight of the adult heart varies with an individual's height and weight. The average weight of the female human heart is 250 to 300 grams; it weighs approximately 300 to 350 grams in men. The heart has four

---

*Most of the information contained in this section is from Vinay Kumar and Abul K. Abbas, *Robbins Pathologic Basis of Disease,* Philadelphia, Penn.: Saunders Elsevier, 1999; and John Hall, *Guyton and Hall Textbook of Medical Physiology,* 11th Edition, Philadelphia, Penn.: Saunders Elsevier, 2010.

chambers: the two upper chambers are called the *atria* (*atrium* in the singular) and the lower two chambers are known as the *ventricles*. Each side of the heart has one atrium and one ventricle. The left and right sides of the heart are separated by a thick septum between the atria, as well as between the ventricles. The diagrammatic features of the human heart are show in figure 2.1.

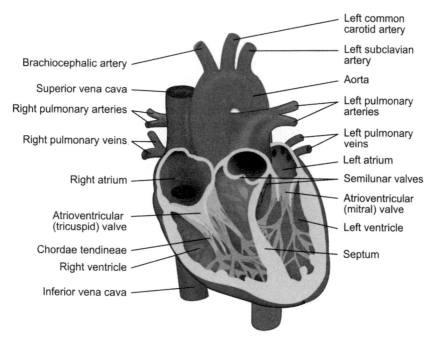

Figure 2.1. The human heart

A series of valves in the human heart allow blood to flow in the correct direction. A function of this is that they also prevent the backflow of blood from one chamber of the heart to another. The tricuspid valve separates the right atrium from the right ventricle. The mitral valve separates the left atrium from the left ventricle. The pulmonary valve separates the right ventricle from the pulmonary arteries. The aortic valve separates the left atrium from the ascending aorta.

The left ventricle of the heart connects with the large main artery called the aorta, which carries blood to various tissues through a series of medium, small, and fine arteries (capillaries). The heart is connected to the lungs through large arteries called pulmonary arteries, which carry deoxygenated blood to the lungs. The lungs send oxygenated blood back to the heart through the pulmonary veins.

PHYSIOLOGY

The adult heart muscle contracts and relaxes at the rate of about seventy to eighty times per minute; it is a never-ceasing pump. This phenomenon is called the heartbeat. Contraction of the heart is referred to as *systole* and relaxation of the heart is called *diastole*. When the ventricles of the heart contract, blood is squeezed into blood vessels leading to the lungs. During the diastolic process, the ventricles of the heart relax, filling the left atria and the right atria with blood.

The adult heart beats about one hundred thousand times a day or about three billion times during a seventy-year period. When an adult heart contracts, it pumps blood through its chambers to the blood vessels of the body, which deliver blood to various tissues. The amount of blood that the heart pumps daily in this fashion is approximately two thousand gallons. During running or (extensive) aerobic exercise, the heart pumps out blood at a faster rate in order to meet the increased demand for oxygen by the body's tissues. However, during sleep or a resting period, the heart pumps out blood more slowly (causing slower heartbeats). Nerves connected to the heart muscle regulate the rate of the heartbeat.

Oxygen is needed for our survival and the proper functioning of our various cells and organs. Blood is oxygenated in the lungs and deoxygenated in the various tissues. Oxygenated blood from the lungs goes to the heart, to the tissues, and to the organs through the arteries. When it reaches the heart, the oxygenated blood enters the left atrium from the right and left pulmonary veins. Oxygenated blood leaves the left ventricle by the ascending aorta, which takes blood to various parts of the body through a complex network of arteries.

Deoxygenated blood from the tissues is carried out through the veins to the heart and then sent to the lungs through the pulmonary arteries. Deoxygenated blood from the tissues enters the right atrium from the superior vena cava and inferior vena cava, and leaves the right ventricle by the pulmonary artery, which takes blood to the lungs through the right and left branches of the pulmonary artery. The diagrammatic representation of oxygenated and deoxygenated blood is described here in a simplified manner.

Deoxygenated blood from tissues ⟶ Major veins ⟶
Right atrium ⟶ Right ventricle ⟶
Pulmonary artery ⟶ Lungs ⟶ Oxygenated blood from lungs ⟶
Pulmonary veins ⟶ Left atrium ⟶ Left ventricle ⟶ Aorta ⟶ Tissues

The nerve cells associated with the heart muscle cells act like electrical wiring to conduct electrical impulses that regulate the contraction and relaxation of the ventricles in a precise, coordinated rhythm, which keeps blood circulating throughout the body in a steady and consistent manner.

DEVELOPMENT

The first physical sign that the heart is developing as an organ occurs sixteen to eighteen days after conception. In its early development, the heart appears as a tube. The heartbeat begins in the third week (following conception), but blood doesn't begin to circulate until the fifth week. During the fourth week, a single large ventricle and the partly separated left and right atrium have developed. By the seventh week, the two ventricles and atria are separated, and the heart is fully developed.

After birth infants need an increased amount of oxygen due to the rapid growth of their body's organs. Thus, the heart's rate of pumping oxygen-rich blood is the most rapid during infancy—about 120 beats per minute. (This heartbeat subsequently slows as the body develops.) The heartbeat of a seven-year-old child is approximately 90 beats per minute. It is about 70 to 80 beats per minute in young adults ages eighteen and older.

RISK FACTORS FOR HEART DISEASE

Heart disease is a complex disease that develops slowly and occurs primarily in older individuals over the age of sixty. Individuals with a family history, however, may develop signs of it when they are under the age of fifty. Let's take a look at some of its causes, risk factors, and the degree to which family history may have a bearing on its onset.

Risk factors for heart disease are those variables that increase one's likelihood of developing the disease. Several external and internal risk factors have been identified. External risk factors include issues related to one's environment, diet, and lifestyle. Internal risk factors include increased oxidative stress and chronic inflammation, high LDL cholesterol, the presence of small lipoprotein particles, triglycerides, low HDL cholesterol, increased homocysteine levels, and high blood pressure. Some risk factors that contribute to the potential for developing heart disease cannot be acted upon, while others can. Let's look at both groups here, beginning with factors that we cannot change.

Inalterable Risk Factors

Age: The risk of developing heart disease increases as we age.

Ethnicity: African American, Hispanic, Native American, Hawaiian, and some Asian American populations have a higher risk of developing heart disease than their Caucasian counterparts do.

Gender: Men have a higher risk of developing heart disease than do women of reproductive age. Men and postmenopausal women, however, share the same risk of its development.

Gene defects (family history): If one's parents had heart disease, the risk of it increases among their children, although it is not a foregone conclusion that if one or both of one's parents had heart disease, their child will develop it as well. This is due to the fact that the genetic defects responsible for increasing the risk of heart disease of the parents are transmitted to some but not to all of their children.

Alterable Risk Factors

Risk factors for developing heart disease that *can* be changed include the following:

Chronic inflammation: Chronic inflammation is a prolonged state that persists following injury and/or infection. It is marked by the presence of lymphocytes and macrophages, an increased number of blood vessels, fibrosis, and the death of the related tissue.

Diabetes: Heart disease and diabetes are two distinct diseases with respect to target organs (heart disease obviously involves the heart and diabetes involves the pancreas). Both diseases impair blood-vessel activity, and some causative agents—such as obesity, physical inactivity, increased oxidative stress, and chronic inflammation—are common to both heart disease and diabetes. Individuals with diabetes have a higher risk of developing heart disease than those who do not have diabetes.

High blood pressure: High blood pressure, if not controlled, can lead to an increased risk of developing heart disease and stroke.

High LDL cholesterol, small lipoprotein particles, triglycerides, and low HDL cholesterol: These abnormal lipid (fat) profiles can increase the risk of heart disease in some individuals. To understand what is meant by this, we need to know what constitutes a normal value and an abnormal one. In terms of total cholesterol, blood levels of 150 mg/dL or lower are considered normal; 150–199 mg/dL is borderline high; 200–249 mg/dL is high; and above 300 mg/dL is considered very high with respect to the risk of heart disease. The higher the value of total cholesterol, the greater is the risk of this disease in some individuals.

In terms of high-density lipoprotein (HDL) cholesterol, a blood level of 40 mg/dL or lower is considered low, and 60 mg/dL or higher is considered high. The higher the level of HDL, the lesser is the risk of this disease in some individuals.

In terms of low-density lipoprotein (LDL) cholesterol, a blood level of 100 mg/dL or lower is normal; 100–129 mg/dL is near normal; 130–159 mg/dL is borderline high; 160–189 mg/dL is high; and 190 mg/dL or above is very high with respect to heart disease. The higher the value of LDL cholesterol, the greater is the risk of this disease in some individuals.

In terms of triglycerides, a blood level lower than 150 mg/dL is considered normal. The higher the value of triglycerides, the greater is the risk of developing heart disease.

Increased homocysteine levels: Homocysteine is a naturally occurring substance that is produced when the amino acids methione and cysteine are broken down. Homocysteine damages endothelial cells by generating excessive amounts of free radicals (Perez-de-Arce et al. 2005). Increased homocysteine levels enhance the risk of heart disease, independent of abnormal changes in lipid profiles in some individuals, by damaging the endothelial cells lining the blood vessels that supply blood to the heart. This means that increased homocysteine may increase the risk of heart disease in the presence of normal lipid profiles (cholesterols and other lipoproteins).

Increased C-reactive protein (CRP) levels: CRP is one of the protein markers of inflammation present in the blood; it is elevated in heart disease. Increased levels of CRP can cause damage to endothelial cells lining the blood vessels and, thus, can increase the risk of developing heart disease in some individuals.

Obesity: It is now established that obesity markedly increases one's risk of developing heart disease.

Oxidative stress: Oxidative stress is a condition in which the increased production of free radicals derived from oxygen and nitrogen occurs. It has been determined that oxidative stress is a contributing factor to heart disease.

Physical inactivity: Persons who perform very little physical activity have a higher risk of developing heart disease than those who are active.

Plaque: The presence of plaque in the arteries makes them stiff and causes a progressive narrowing of them, which can reduce or even stop the blood supply. This contributes to an elevated risk of heart disease.

Smoking of tobacco: The smoking of tobacco is one of the major lifestyle-related factors that increases the risk of developing heart disease in both men and women.

A CLOSER LOOK
AT SOME RISK FACTORS

As discussed we can impact some of the risk factors previously discussed so as to mitigate the negative ramifications of heart disease. Other variables are inalterable. Let's look at some of these variables in greater detail here, beginning with the factors that we cannot change: the effects of aging on the development of heart disease and the role that family history may play in its onset.

Aging
An increased production of free radicals contributes to the aging process. Excessive amounts of free radicals are produced by mitochondria, which are present in abundance in heart muscle cells. Unfortunately, mitochondria are very vulnerable to damage produced by free radicals. This is primarily due to the fact that the DNA that is present in mitochondria

is not protected by protein and therefore is easily damaged. The damaged mitochondria consequently produce more free radicals and less energy, which increases the risk of heart disease. Increased levels of oxidized proteins (proteins damaged by free radicals) and mutations in the DNA of mitochondria are found in an aging mouse model (premature aging), which closely resembles age-related changes in the human heart. These effects of aging in mice are prevented by overexpressing the antioxidant enzyme catalase, which is targeted to mitochondria (Dai and Rabinovitch 2009).

During aging a loss of muscle mass occurs. One of the reasons for this is that oxidized proteins (proteins damaged by free radicals) are not removed from the body. Proteasomes, which constitute a complex enzyme system present in all cells, are responsible for removing damaged proteins, but they fail do so as the body ages because the increased burden of free radicals has damaged them and rendered them less effective in this regard (Davies and Shringarpure 2006). Damaged proteasomes can thus be the cause of an increase in the accumulation of oxidized proteins in the cells, which eventually kill the cells.

A normal length of a telomere, a part of a chromosome, is essential for maintaining the ability of cells to perform their functions in all of the body's organs. During aging the length of the chromosome's telomeres gradually decreases. Increased oxidative stress causes the telomeres to shorten more quickly. This is supported by the fact that dietary antioxidants such as vitamins C and E reduce the rate of telomere-shortening (Tanaka et al. 2007).

The effectiveness of some antioxidants such as vitamin E, glutathione, and coenzyme Q10 decreases as we age. The reduced potency of these antioxidants serves to increase the level of oxidative stress in the body.*

Thus, although we have demonstrated the effects of aging on the

---

*This issue has been examined in greater detail in K. N. Prasad and K. C. Prasad, *Fighting Cancer with Vitamins and Antioxidants: A Guide to Prevention and Treatment*, Rochester, Vt.: Healing Arts Press, 2011.

development of heart disease, we should also know that recent scientific studies suggest that younger people are showing earlier signs of heart disease because of an increasing incidence of obesity and physical inactivity in this demographic.

Cholesterol

Cholesterol plays a part in the initiation and progression of heart disease. However, about 50 percent of patients who are hospitalized with symptoms of a heart attack have normal cholesterol levels (Hecht and Superko 2001). Nevertheless, improving cholesterol profiles is considered one of the more effective strategies that an individual can pursue to reduce the risk of developing heart disease.

Cholesterols are formed from dietary fats or are made in the liver. The formation of different types of cholesterol from dietary fats is a very complex process. Therefore, it is presented here in simplified form. Dietary fats are not soluble in water; therefore, they cannot be absorbed from the intestine. For this reason fats are initially solubilized in the intestine with the help of bile salts secreted from the gallbladder and enzymes called lipoprotein lipases that are secreted from the pancreas.

These pancreatic enzymes convert solubilized fats into free fatty acids that enter the intestinal cells, where they form triacylglycerols and cholesterols. Triacylglycerols and cholesterols formed from dietary fats, as well as those made in the liver, combine with proteins to form lipid-protein complexes (lipoproteins). These lipoproteins vary in their lipid and protein content and they contain cholesterols, which can be in very low-density lipid (VLDL) form, low-density lipid (LDL) form, or high-density lipid (HDL) form.

In the blood VLDLs are converted to LDLs by the action of lipoprotein lipase enzymes. LDLs are the carriers of cholesterols to various tissues in the body. HDLs consist of lipids and proteins of different sizes and form in the liver and small intestine. HDL also contains different forms of apoproteins (apoA-1, apoC-1, apoC-II, and apoE). ApoA-1s represent 70 percent of all apoproteins. In the early stages of its formation,

HDL lacks cholesterols, which it soon acquires from the peripheral tissues. One of the major functions of HDL is to transport acquired cholesterols back to the liver, where they are converted to bile acid and then stored in the gallbladder. In addition to apoproteins, HDL also contains many enzymes, including the antioxidant enzyme glutathione peroxidase. HDL exhibits antioxidant and anti-inflammatory activities.

Family History

Now let's examine the role that a family history of heart disease may play in its development. If the gene defects of heart disease pass from one generation to another, the development of heart disease in a child can be attributed to a family history of this disease. However, it may otherwise be difficult to ascertain whether or not heart disease is due to one's family history or whether its onset is due to lifestyle and dietary choices that have catalyzed its development. Suppose that one or both parents were smokers or had other risk factors for developing heart disease and died of heart attack at the age of seventy or older. Does this mean that their children would inherit the genes responsible for increasing their chances of developing heart disease? The answer is no.

Generally, individuals who derive from a family with a history of heart disease are not impacted by the lifestyle and dietary choices that their forebears made. What *is* true is that they (the children) are at increased risk of developing heart disease at a younger age if their parents died young (under the age of fifty) of the disease. In both men and women, family history of heart disease is a strong and independent risk factor for its development (Leander et al. 2001). The gene defects responsible for increasing the risk of developing heart disease interact with other risk factors in a synergistic manner (more than that produced by gene defects or environmental agents alone). The individual with a family history of heart disease should avoid exacerbating the prevalent risk factors as much as possible, and should instead make wise and prudent choices in regard to lifestyle and dietary considerations.

Let's now turn our attention to how some of the factors that we *are* capable of influencing may impact our chances of developing heart disease.

Obesity

Studies done on mice to date have formed the general discussion regarding factors that impact the development of heart disease. Feeding apoE-deficient mice a high-fat diet increased their levels of pro-inflammatory cytokines. These cytokines included interleukin-6 (IL-6), tumor necrosis factor-alpha (TNF-alpha), and markers of oxidative damage in vascular smooth muscle cells. These pro-inflammatory cytokines play a primary role in the initiation and progression of atherosclerosis and heart disease. An infusion of the insulin-like growth factor-1 (IGF-1) decreased levels of pro-inflammatory cytokines and markers of oxidative damage, as well as the progression of atherosclerosis and plaque (Sukhanov et al. 2007).

Mice fed with a high-fat, high-sugar diet displayed a progressive increase in the size of their left ventricle, which caused a reduced pumping of blood. These animals had elevated levels of markers of oxidative damage. These animals also had increased levels of plasma glucose and showed insulin resistance. Treatment with resveratrol, an antioxidant isolated from grape seeds, prevented damage to the heart in these mice (Qin et al. 2012).

It was found that obesity also increased the risk of atrial fibrillation by dilating the left atrial (Wang and Parise et al. 2004). This effect of obesity is due to an increased production of free radicals.

While studying the development of heart disease in a genetic model of mice (transgenic mice), it was found that the activity of the enzyme cytochrome P450 2E1 (CYP2E1) increases. This enzyme activity is responsible for producing free radicals (Zhang et al. 2011).

Plaque

It is thought that plaque, especially unstable plaque, plays a central role in precipitating heart attacks and strokes. Plaque is a fatlike substance found in the walls of veins and arteries of the body. Plaque buildup may cause a narrowing of the coronary arteries that supply blood to the heart. If these vital arteries are injured, platelet aggregation may occur within the wall of the artery adjacent to the plaque. However, if the plaque ruptures, a blood clot can form on the surface of the artery. Depending on the size of the clot, the blood flow to the heart can be partially or fully blocked. Sometime clots may also break free, causing a blockage of blood that supplies distant organs such as the brain, which can cause a stroke. Clots may also block the blood vessels to the lungs, which may lead to death.

It's important to understand how plaque is formed. LDL cholesterol is commonly referred to as "bad cholesterol" because high LDL cholesterol levels are associated with an increased risk of developing heart disease. However, it's the *oxidized* form of LDL cholesterol (cholesterol that has been damaged by free radicals) that increases the risk of developing heart disease.

LDL cholesterol is easily oxidized (damaged) by free radicals, and as we've stated oxidized LDL cholesterol may be one of the early events initiating plaque formation. It does this in several ways: by enhancing platelet adhesion and aggregation; by impairing the elasticity of the coronary arteries (Holvoet and Collen 1994); by triggering thrombosis (clot formation); and by increasing the formation of foam cells (cells filled with tiny bubbles).

Oxidized LDL cholesterol is engulfed by macrophages to form foam cells. C-reactive protein (CRP, a marker of chronic inflammation), increases the uptake of oxidized LDL cholesterol by macrophages and thereby increases the number of foam cells (Becker et al. 2001).

Oxidized LDL cholesterol can also increase the proliferation of vascular smooth muscle cells by activating the c-Myc cellular gene (de Nigris et al. 2000). Both foam cells and the increased proliferation of vascular smooth muscle cells contribute to the formation of plaque in coronary arteries.

Once plaque is formed, it serves as a continuous stimulus for increased inflammatory reactions that release reactive oxygen species (ROS; free radicals derived from oxygen) and pro-inflammatory cytokines, all of which are toxic to heart cells. Oxidized LDL cholesterol also significantly enhances the TNF-alpha-stimulated production of reactive oxygen species and the endothelial adhesiveness of monocyte/mononuclear cells.

Thus we see how an increase in oxidative stress contributes to atherosclerosis (Chen et al. 2006). These studies suggest that lowering the level of LDL cholesterol and preventing its oxidation should reduce the risk of developing plaque and atherosclerosis.

Endothelial cells line the walls of the blood vessels that supply blood to the heart. Endothelial cells of the vascular wall are damaged by free radicals. They are also damaged by products that are released from chronic inflammatory reactions and homocysteine. It's now recognized that endothelial cell dysfunction may also be one of the early events in the development of heart disease (Drexler 1999). Damaged endothelial cells may reduce the activity of nitric oxide synthase (NOS), an enzyme responsible for making nitric oxide (NO), which would decrease the production of NO. Since NO regulates dilation of blood vessels, a reduction in NO would reduce the dilation of blood vessels.

It should be mentioned that an excessive production of NO may also be harmful. This is due to the fact that the oxidation of NO forms peroxynitrite, a form of free radical that can cause damage to the arteries, causing dysfunction. Thus, in order to maintain the normal functioning of blood vessels, it is essential to maintain the proper levels of NO in the body. Both deficiency and excess production of NO can impair blood-vessel activity and enhance endothelial dysfunction. Therefore, protecting the endothelial cells against free radical damage and preventing the formation of plaque may be considered useful strategies in reducing the risk of developing heart disease.

A diagrammatic representation of plaque formation is illustrated in figure 2.2 on page 28.

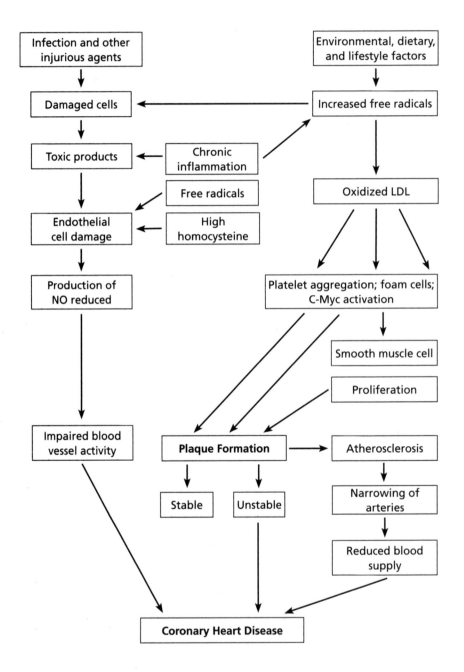

*Figure 2.2. Diagrammatic Representation of
Major Biochemical Steps That Contribute
to the Formation of Plaque*

The Smoking of Tobacco

The smoking of tobacco increases the levels of nitric oxide in the body, and generates other forms of free radicals. It also depletes antioxidant levels in the body (Duthie et al. 1991; Reznick et al. 1992). Additionally, an excessive production of nitric oxide can form peroxynitrite, a nitrogen-derived free radical, which is highly damaging.

The smoking of tobacco is also associated with an increased blood concentration of C-reactive protein (a marker of chronic inflammation) in men and women. It was found that the CRP levels of older men and women who had quit smoking returned to normal after several years of abstinence from tobacco (Dietrich et al. 2007).

CONCLUDING REMARKS

The human heart is one of the major organs of the body and is essentially a muscular pump that propels and expels blood through its chambers, beating roughly seventy-two times per minute in the healthy adult. It pumps oxygen and glucose to the brain, helping it to maintain consciousness, and it pumps the proper combinations of sodium, calcium, and potassium salts, as well as oxygen, glucose, and amino acids, to the muscles. Our glands and tissues likewise need many of these raw materials in order to be able to function properly.

Nerves connected to the heart muscle regulate the rate of the heartbeat, which keeps the blood pumping in a steady, rhythmic manner. Blood is oxygenated in the lungs and deoxygenated in the various tissues of the body. Oxygenated blood from the lungs is carried to the tissues and organs through the arteries, and deoxygenated blood from the tissues is carried through the veins to the heart and then to the lungs for oxygenation.

There are several risk factors that increase the chance of developing heart disease, some of which cannot be acted upon for mitigation, some of which can. Family history is a significant factor that one cannot influence. If a male in your immediate family has had a heart attack before the age of fifty-five, or if a female in your immediate family has had one before the age of sixty-five, you are at a greater risk of developing heart disease yourself. Similarly if both parents, prior to the age of fifty-five, have developed heart disease, one's risk of developing it can be as high as 50 percent when compared to a normal baseline population. Other risk factors that cannot be changed include the variables of age, gender, and ethnicity.

Even if one has a family history of heart disease, and especially if this is so, it becomes necessary to try to mitigate other risk factors that *can* be controlled. These risk factors include obesity, physical inactivity, high blood pressure, high LDL cholesterol, the smoking of tobacco, drug abuse, increased oxidative stress, chronic inflammation, and elevated homocysteine levels. Again one can institute some fundamental lifestyle changes and adaptations to protect the heart. These include the incorporation of moderate exercise into your daily routine, being mindful of the fat and salt content of the food you eat and making the necessary adjustments, and dieting in a sensible manner to bring your weight down, should you be overweight or obese.

There are other strategies that can be employed to protect oneself against the crippling ramifications of heart disease. We will be discussing them in the ensuing chapters of this book.

3 Compounding Factors of Heart Disease

Oxidative Stress and Inflammation

Before exploring the issues of prevention and the improved treatment of heart disease, it would behoove us to become familiar with oxidative stress and the process of inflammation, which play key roles in the development of cardiac issues and concerns. It is equally essential that we become familiar with free radicals—which contribute to oxidative stress—and antioxidants—which are vital in protecting against oxidative stress and inflammation. In this chapter we will examine these topics.

OXIDATIVE STRESS

Oxidative stress (also referred to as oxidative damage) occurs in the body when the levels of free radicals exceed the body's antioxidant capacity to neutralize them. What are free radicals? They are atoms, molecules, or ions with unpaired electrons, derived from either oxygen or nitrogen. In 1900 the first organic free radical, triphenylmethyl radical, was identified by Moses Gomberg of the University of Michigan. Free radicals are symbolized by a dot "•".

Free radicals can damage all cellular structures, including deoxyribonucleic acid (DNA), ribonucleic acid (RNA), proteins, fats, and membranes. Our body produces different types of free radicals, most of which are very short-lived; their half-lives* vary from 10^{-9} seconds to days. This means that most of them are quickly destroyed after causing damage. Here are some examples of them and their half-lives:

Half-Lives of Some Free Radicals

Hydroxyl = 10^{-9} seconds

Superoxide anion = 10^{-5} seconds

Nitric oxide = about 1 second

Lipid peroxyl = 7 seconds

Hydrogen peroxide = minutes

Semiquinone = days

Sources of increased oxidative stress† include:

1. Aging (wherein the reduced antioxidant capacity of the body allows for increased oxidative stress)
2. Damage to mitochondria (wherein the reduced use of oxygen generates excessive amounts of free radicals)
3. High glucose levels (as found in diabetes)
4. Increased levels of free iron and copper in the blood (free iron is iron that is not bound to any protein)
5. Increased utilization of oxygen (generates excessive amounts of free radicals)

---

*A half-life is the amount of time required for a quantity to fall to half its value as measured at the beginning of the time period.

†The reader will note that some of the sources of oxidative stress that are listed have been noted in the previous chapter as being factors we can alter to mitigate heart disease.

6. Obesity (can cause insulin resistance, which increases blood glucose levels)

7. The smoking of tobacco (depletes antioxidants and generates free radicals)

Oxidation and Reduction Processes

To fully understand the role that free radicals and antioxidants play, it is beneficial to grasp the relationship between the processes of oxidation and reduction that are constantly taking place in the body. It is also helpful to understand the processes that produce free radicals.

Oxidation is a process by which an atom or a molecule gains oxygen, loses hydrogen, or loses an electron. For example, carbon gains oxygen during oxidation and becomes carbon dioxide. A superoxide radical loses an electron during the oxidation process and becomes oxygen. Thus, an *oxidizing agent* is an atom or molecule that changes another chemical by adding oxygen to it or by removing an electron or hydrogen from it. Examples of oxidizing agents include free radicals, X-rays, and ozone.

Reduction is a process by which an atom or molecule loses oxygen, gains hydrogen, or gains an electron. For example, carbon dioxide loses oxygen and becomes carbon monoxide, carbon gains hydrogen and becomes methane, and oxygen gains an electron and becomes a superoxide anion. Thus, a *reducing agent* is an atom or molecule that changes another chemical by removing oxygen from it or by adding an electron or hydrogen to it.

All antioxidants may be considered reducing agents. If the body's internal environment is inclined to the process of reduction (versus oxidation), the risk of developing chronic diseases—including heart disease—may be decreased. The reduction process would be favored if and when an elevated level of antioxidants exists (with the exception of an elevated level of oxidized antioxidants). Oxidized antioxidants, having been damaged by free radicals, act as a prooxidants—like a free radical—rather than as antioxidants.

Oxidative stress, as we have learned, refers to a condition in which the increased production of free radicals derived from oxygen occurs. *Nitrosylative stress* refers to a condition in which the increased production of free radicals derived from nitrogen occurs. Both increased oxidative stress and nitrosylative stress increase the risk of chronic disease.

Processes Involving Oxygen and Nitrogen in the Production of Free Radicals

The formative process of some reactive oxygen species (ROS: free radicals derived from oxygen) is described below.

When molecular oxygen (O_2) acquires an electron, the superoxide anion ($O_2^{\bullet-}$) is formed:

$$O_2 + e^- = O_2^{\bullet-}$$

Superoxide dismutase (SOD) and H^+ can react with $O_2^{\bullet-}$ to form hydrogen peroxide (H_2O_2):

$$2O_2^{\bullet-} + 2H^+ \text{ plus SOD} \rightarrow H_2O_2 + O_2$$
$$O_2^{\bullet-} + H^+ \rightarrow HO_2^{\bullet} \text{ (hydroperoxy radical)}$$
$$2HO_2^{\bullet} \rightarrow H_2O_2 + O_2$$

Ferric and ferrous forms of iron can react with superoxide anion and hydrogen peroxide to produce molecular oxygen (O_2) and hydroxyl radicals ($OH^{\bullet}$), respectively:

$$Fe^{3+} + O_2^{\bullet-} \rightarrow Fe^{2+} + O_2$$
$$Fe_2^+ + H_2O_2 \rightarrow Fe^{3+} + OH^{\bullet} + OH^- \text{ (Fenton reaction)}$$

Hydroxyl radicals can also be formed from superoxide anion by the Haber-Weiss reaction:

$$O_2^{\bullet-} + H_2O_2 \rightarrow O_2 + OH^- + OH^{\bullet}$$

Both the Fenton and Haber-Weiss reactions require a transition metal such as copper or iron. Among ROS, OH$^\bullet$ is the most damaging free radical and is very short-lived.

Hydroxyl radicals are very reactive with a variety of organic compounds, leading to the production of more radical compounds:

$$RH \text{ (organic compound)} + OH^\bullet \rightarrow R^\bullet \text{ (organic radical)} + H_2O$$
$$R^\bullet + O_2 \rightarrow RO_2^\bullet \text{ (peroxyl radical)}$$

For example, the DNA radical can be generated by reaction with a hydroxyl radical, and this can lead to a break in the DNA strand.

Catalase detoxifies hydrogen peroxide to form water and molecular oxygen:

$$H_2O_2 + \text{catalase} \rightarrow H_2O \text{ and } O_2$$

Reactive nitrogen species (RNS: free radicals derived from nitrogen) are represented by nitric oxide (NO$^\bullet$). NO is synthesized by the enzyme nitric oxide synthase from L-arginine. NO$^\bullet$ can combine with superoxide anion to form peroxynitrite, a powerful oxidant.

$$NO^\bullet + O_2^{\bullet-} \rightarrow ONOO^- \text{ (peroxynitrite)}$$

When protonated (likely at physiological pH), peroxynitrite spontaneously decomposes to reactive nitric dioxide and hydroxyl radicals:

$$ONOO^- + H^+ \rightarrow {}^\bullet NO_2 + OH^\bullet$$

Superoxide dismutase (SOD) can also enhance the peroxynitrite-mediated nitration of tyrosine residues on critical proteins, presumably via species similar to the nitronium cation (NO$_2^+$):

$$ONOO^- \text{ plus SOD} \rightarrow NO_2 + \rightarrow \text{Nitration of tyrosine}$$

Processes That Produce Free Radicals

Free radicals are created during the intake of oxygen, in the course of infection, and during the oxidative metabolism of certain compounds.

Mitochondria are the major sites where free radicals are produced. They are elongated membranous structures in the cells and are responsible for producing energy. While generating energy with the help of oxygen, mitochondria produce certain types of free radicals (superoxide anions and hydroxyl radicals) as by-products. During this process about 2 percent of unused oxygen leaks out of the mitochondria and makes about 20 billion molecules of superoxide anions and hydrogen peroxide per cell per day.

During a bacterial or viral infection, phagocytic cells (a kind of white blood cell) engulf invading microorganisms and generate high levels of nitric oxide, superoxide anions, and hydrogen peroxide in order to kill the infectious organisms. The excessive production of free radicals by phagocytes can damage normal cells. Free radicals are also produced in the course of the metabolism of fatty acids and other molecules in the body. Certain habits such as tobacco smoking and the absorption of some trace minerals such as free iron, copper, and manganese can increase the rate of free-radical production. In this manner the human body is constantly exposed to different types and varying levels of free radicals. Fortunately, we have antioxidant defense systems that protect the body against free-radical damage.

The Effect of Free Radicals on the Heart

As we have learned, free radicals are generated primarily in the mitochondria, which utilize oxygen to generate energy for the body. Therefore an organ such as the heart, which has an abundance of mitochondria, is very vulnerable to oxidative damage. Mitochondria in the heart cells are also easily damaged by free radicals because mitochondrial DNA is not protected by proteins. This is in contrast to the DNA in the nucleus of a cell, which *is* protected by proteins. In the case of the heart, damaged mitochondria produce reduced amounts of energy, thereby decreasing the ability of heart muscle cells to function properly.

It has been demonstrated that the activity of the enzyme xanthine oxidase, which is responsible for the production of free radicals, is elevated in heart disease (Bergamini et al. 2009). An elevated activity of this enzyme would increase the production of free radicals, which can cause cardiac hypertrophy (an increase in the size of the heart), myocardial fibrosis (wherein muscle cells are replaced by fibroblasts), and a blood-pumping defect of the left ventricle.

Increased levels of norepinephrine, which occur during stress, enhanced the production of free radicals. Treatment with n-acetylcysteine blocked the effect of norepinephrine on the production of free radicals (Xiong et al. 2012).

Hypoxia (a reduction in the amount of available oxygen), which causes ischemic heart disease, also produces excessive amounts of free radicals. This effect of hypoxia is mitigated by the suppression of protein kinase C epsilon (PKCέ) (Patterson et al. 2012). Controlled activation of PCKέ protects against ischemic heart disease, whereas uncontrolled chronic activation may increase the risk of diabetes and cancer.

Carnitine deficiency is a genetic disease that may increase the risk of heart disease and ventricular fibrillation. Increased levels of markers of oxidative damage, such as reactive aldehyde-4-hydroxy-2-nonenal, a product of lipid peroxidation, were found in a patient with carnitine deficiency (Mazzini et al. 2011).

Following an injury to myocardium, the heart undergoes remodeling (changes in size, shape, structure, and function) in order to prevent heart attack. Increased oxidative stress can cause abnormal heart remodeling, which can increase the risk of heart failure (Sirker et al. 2007).

Chronic damage to the heart cells by free radicals can initiate chronic inflammation, which produces toxic chemicals. Thus, increased oxidative stress and chronic inflammation play a key role in the development and progression of heart disease (Tsutsui et al. 2011).

It has also been reported that two contractile proteins of the left ventricle—actin and tropomyosin—are damaged by free radicals during an early phase of heart failure, suggesting that increased oxidative damage may contribute to the malfunction of a ventricle (Canton et al. 2011).

INFLAMMATION

Inflammation in Latin is referred to as *inflammare,* or "setting on fire." The primary features of inflammation (at affected sites) include redness, swelling, warmth, and varying degrees of pain. These characteristics of inflammation were first recognized by the renowned Roman medical scholar, Aulus Cornelius Celsus, (circa 25 BCE to 50 CE).

Injury to cells initiates inflammation. This cell injury may be caused by physical agents such as radiation, chemical toxins, mechanical trauma, or infection. Inflammation is generally considered a protective response. However, it can also act as a double-edged sword. Inflammation is needed to kill harmful invading organisms and for the removal of cellular debris in order to facilitate the recovery process at the site of injury, but inflammation can also damage normal tissues by releasing a number of toxic chemicals.

In any event inflammation is a highly complex biological response that is tightly regulated and automatically turned off after the recovery process is complete. During the healing process, the injured tissue is replaced by a regeneration of original cell type. Or the injured site is filled in with fibroblastic tissue (scarring). Most commonly, the healing that takes place is a combination of both processes. If the damage is not repaired, a chronic inflammatory response is set in motion. Chronic inflammation is associated with most chronic diseases, including heart disease.

Inflammation is divided into two categories: acute and chronic.

Acute Inflammation

Acute inflammation occurs following cellular injury or infection with microorganisms. The period of acute inflammation is fairly short, typically lasting from a few minutes to a few days. Acute inflammation occurs soon after an individual has suffered an injury. It participates in the successful healing of the injury when tissue damage is not severe. If the tissue damage is extensive, acute inflammatory reactions continue. The toxic products released during acute inflammation may contribute to organ failure and eventually even death.

Chronic Inflammation

Chronic inflammation occurs following persistent cellular injury and infection. The period of chronic inflammation is relatively long and may last for the duration of the injury or infection. The main features of chronic inflammation are the presence of an increased number of lymphocytes and macrophages, the proliferation of blood vessels, fibrosis (an extensive proliferation of fibroblasts), and tissue death.

In addition to causing increased oxidative stress, chronic inflammation plays a role in the initiation and progression of heart disease and atherosclerosis. Chronic inflammation may be caused by damage to endothelial cells by free radicals. It may also be caused by infective agents such as bacteria—Chlamydia pneumonia and Helicobacter pylori for instance—and viruses that include herpes simplex and cytomegalovirus.

During chronic inflammation, several highly toxic agents are released. They include:

1. Adhesion molecules
2. Complement proteins
3. C-reactive proteins (CRP)
4. Cytokines (pro-inflammatory and anti-inflammatory)
5. Eicosanoids (arachidonic acid metabolites)
6. Reactive oxygen species (ROS; free radicals derived from oxygen)

Let's examine these toxic agents in a bit more detail now.

Adhesion Molecules

Adhesion molecules are sticky cell surface proteins that facilitate binding and communication between cells. They are called cell adhesion molecules (CAMs), and they are essential for the development and growth of fetuses. They also participate in inflammatory processes and wound-healing. Although CAMs are essential for the normal development and functioning of the blood vessels, their elevated levels have been implicated in the initiation and progression of various forms of heart disease. There are three major types of CAMs; they are listed here.

1. Immunoglobulin molecules
2. Integrins
3. Selectins

Immunoglobulin molecules: There are three major forms of immunoglobulin molecules: intercellular adhesion molecules (ICAM-1, -2, and -3), vascular cell adhesion molecule-1 (VCAM-1), and platelet endothelial cell adhesion molecule-1 (PECAM-1).

ICAM-1 and -2 are found in endothelial cells, lymphocytes, and leukocytes. They help in the migration of leukocytes at the site of inflammation in endothelial cells. ICAM-3 also plays an important role in leukocyte intercellular interactions.

VCAM-1 is found in large amounts on the surface of endothelial cells activated by pro-inflammatory cytokines (Golias et al. 2007), and it helps to secure leukocytes that are bound to the walls of blood vessels.

PECAM-1 regulates the migration of leukocytes between endothelial cells, and promotes the release of protease enzymes from the neutrophils. Increased levels of immunoglobulin molecules contribute to blood-vessel damage.

Integrins: Integrins facilitate cell-cell binding and the adhesion of cells to an extracellular protein matrix such as collagen or fibronectin (Hillis and Flapan 1998). Increased levels of integrins may also increase platelet aggregation, which increases the risk of heart disease.

Selectins: Selectins recruit leukocytes to the endothelium cells during inflammation, which contributes to the formation of plaque.

Complement Proteins

Complement proteins are essential for a proper functioning of the immune system. The blood contains more than thirty complement proteins, including degradation products, which help immune cells fight infection in the following ways:

1. They enhance phagocytic activity (the engulfing ability) of macrophages
2. They attract macrophages and neutrophils by inducing inflammation in order to kill invading bacteria or viruses
3. They rupture the membranes of invading infectious agents such as bacteria and viruses

Complement proteins are made primarily in liver cells, but are also made by the immune system (macrophages and monocytes). Cells of other organs such as the heart and the intestine also make these proteins. Complement proteins are numbered C-1 through C-9, each of which has a complex mechanism of action on cells.

Although activation of complement proteins is essential for protecting the host against infectious agents such as bacteria and viruses, excessive activation of these proteins may cause inflammation and thereby increase the risk of atherosclerosis and heart disease. Harmful effects of activated complement proteins on the heart are supported by the fact that inhibition of the activation of complement proteins reduced damage to the heart (Aukrust et al. 2001).

Activation of complement proteins plays a role in the development of atherosclerosis (Malik et al. 2010).

Elevated levels of the complement protein C-3 have been found in heart disease (Onat et al. 2010). Because of this it can be used as a marker of heart disease.

C-Reactive Proteins (CRP)

The level of CRP in the blood is considered one of the markers of chronic inflammation. Extensive studies indicate that increased levels of CRP are associated with an increased risk of developing heart disease. For example, a well-designed clinical study of apparently healthy men revealed that those with the highest levels of CRP had a 3-fold increase in their risk of heart disease, and a 2-fold increase in their risk of stroke (Ridker et al. 1997).

In another clinical study, it was found that postmenopausal women who had high levels of CRP had a more than 4-fold increase in the risk of developing heart disease in comparison to those who had low levels of CRP (Ridker et al. 2000).

Others have suggested that increased levels of CRP are only a moderate predictor of heart disease (Danesh et al. 2004).

Studies also exist that suggest increased levels of CRP may *not* be the predictor of heart disease (Danesh and Pepys 2009). However, most studies on how CRP might increase the risk of heart disease have made it very clear that this protein plays a significant role in the development and progression of heart disease.

Treatment with CRP of endothelial cells lining the blood vessels supplying blood to the heart increased the expression of eleven genes and decreased the expression of six genes by more than 2-fold. The IL-18 gene* was elevated by about 13.6-fold in CRP-treated endothelial cells. This increase in IL-18 gene expression was blocked by the anti-IL-18 antibody (Wang et al. 2005).

In high-risk patients with heart disease, the levels of CRP, IL-18, and IL-6 were elevated. Elevated levels of fasting glucose increased the predictive value of IL-18 in heart disease (Troseid et al. 2009).

Treatment with CRP of endothelial cells from blood vessels of the heart increased the plasma levels of matrix metalloproteinase-1 and

---

*The IL-18 gene is a gene for the expression of pro-inflammatory cytokines.

-10 (MMP-1 and MMP-10). Both CRP and MMP-10 are present in advanced plaque (Montero et al. 2006).

Treatment with CRP of endothelial cells of the heart's blood vessels elevated levels of the oxidized LDL receptor-1 (LOX-1), which increased monocyte adhesion to the endothelial cells and uptake of oxidized LDL by monocytes (Li et al. 2004). These changes contribute to the formation of plaque.

Elevated levels of CRP increased platelet adhesion to the endothelial cells of blood vessels. This effect of CRP was mediated by another substance called P-selectin. Platelet adhesion may lead to thrombus (blood clot) formation (Grad et al. 2011). Blood clots can partially or fully block blood flow to the heart, depending on the size of the blood clot. CRP treatment increases levels of the intracellular adhesion molecule-1 (ICAM-1) and the vascular adhesion molecule-1 (VCAM-1), as well as the production and release of the chemokine, monocyte chemoattractant protein-1 (MCP-1).

These effects of CRP cause a migration of monocytes and T-lymphocytes into the walls of blood vessels, thereby promoting atherosclerosis (Pasceri et al. 2001).

In summary high levels of blood CRP may increase the risk of heart disease by the following mechanisms:

1. Causes changes in the expression of several genes
2. Increases production of cytokine interleukin-18 (IL-18), a predictor of heart disease
3. Increases the levels of matrix metalloproteinase-1 and -10 (MMP-1 and MMP-10) that may contribute to plaque formation
4. Enhances the levels of oxidized LDL receptor-1 (LOX-1) that increases the adhesion of monocytes to the endothelial cells of blood vessels supplying blood to the heart
5. Increases platelet adhesion to the endothelial cells that can lead to the formation of thrombus (a blood clot that forms in a blood vessel)

6. Increases the levels of intracellular adhesion molecule-1 (ICAM-1) and vascular adhesion molecule-1 (VCAM-1) and the production and release of the chemokine monocyte chemoattractant protein-1 (MCP-1) that promotes atherosclerosis

The values of blood levels of CRP in relation to the risk of developing heart disease are described in the following table.

TABLE 3.1. THE VALUES OF BLOOD LEVELS OF CRP IN RELATION TO THE RISK OF DEVELOPING HEART DISEASE

Levels of CRP in blood	Risk of heart disease
Less than 1.0 mg/L	Low
1.0–2.9 mg/L	Medium
Greater than 3.0 mg/L	High

Cytokines

Cytokines are small proteins that are made by one cell and act on another. They are produced primarily by activated immune cells, such as lymphocytes and macrophages, and are released during both acute and chronic inflammation. There are two types of cytokines: pro-inflammatory cytokines and anti-inflammatory cytokines. A complex network of cytokines maintains a balance between the effects of pro-inflammatory cytokines and anti-inflammatory cytokines. If this balance is altered in favor of pro-inflammatory cytokines, a chronic disease such as heart disease may develop.

Examples of pro-inflammatory cytokines include interleukin-1 (IL-1), IL-6, IL-8, IL-15, IL-16, IL-17, IL-18, tumor necrosis factor-alpha, TGF-beta, and interferon gamma-. These pro-inflammatory cytokines are toxic to cells. Anti-inflammatory cytokines include IL-4, IL-10, IL-11, and IL-13. These cytokines help to heal damaged areas and are released in response to injury by infection, increased oxidative damage to cells, and physical injury to cells.

Pro-inflammatory cytokines are elevated in heart disease. An elevated level of IL-16, a pro-inflammatory cytokine, was associated with the increased risk of heart disease (Wu et al. 2011).

Some of the markers of pro-inflammatory cytokines are elevated in patients with atrial fibrillation, which is a form of heart disease (Schnabel et al. 2009).

Eicosanoids

Arachidonic acid (AA) is a 20-carbon fatty acid that is derived from dietary sources or is formed from the essential fatty acid linoleic acid. During inflammation AA metabolites, also called eicosanoids, are released. These eicosanoids have diverse biological actions, some of which are beneficial. The eicosanoids themselves, in excessive amounts, are harmful, depending on the cell type being acted on and the type of eicosanoid. Eicosanoids include prostaglandins, thromboxanes, leukotrienes, and lipoxins. The enzyme cyclooxygenase (COX) is responsible for making prostaglandins and thromboxanes, and the enzyme lipooxygenase is responsible for making leukotrienes and lipoxins.

There are different forms of prostaglandins (PGs) and thromboxanes (TXs). Some of them dilate blood vessels and prevent platelet aggregation, and others cause an aggregation of platelets. For example, prostacyclin (PGI2) is a potent dilator of blood vessels and reduces platelet aggregation. In contrast thromboxane A2 (TXA2) causes an aggregation of platelets. Aspirin reduces the formation of both prostaglandins and thromboxanes by inhibiting activity of the COX enzyme.

Reactive Oxygen Species (ROS)

Neopterin is a catabolic product of guanosine triphosphate, a purine nucleotide. It is part of the chemical group known as pteridines. During inflammation neopterin is released by macrophages; therefore, it can be considered to be a marker of inflammation. High blood levels of this marker are associated with the increased production of reactive oxygen species. It has been reported that the serum levels of neopterin were elevated in patients with heart disease, compared to those who had normal levels of neopterin (Murr et al. 2009).

CONCLUDING REMARKS

Free radicals are highly damaging chemicals that are produced in the human body. They are generated during the use of oxygen, in the course of bacterial or viral infection, and in the context of the normal metabolism of certain compounds. There are several types of free radicals in the body; some are derived from oxygen, others are derived from nitrogen. Oxidative stress refers to a condition in which high levels of free radicals are produced, causing damage to the cells. Increased oxidative stress may be one of the more significant factors involved in increasing the risk of developing heart disease and diabetes. Causes of oxidative stress include:

1. Aging
2. Damaged mitochondria
3. During the oxidative metabolism of certain compounds
4. Excessive use of oxygen such as during aerobic exercise
5. Exposure to ionizing radiation such as X-rays
6. Increased levels of free iron and copper
7. Infection
8. Obesity
9. Smoking tobacco

The cell injury that is caused by physical agents such as radiation, free radicals, chemical toxins, mechanical trauma, or infection initiates a biological event called inflammation. Generally a protective response, inflammation can also be detrimental in that it may release toxic chemicals as part of the inflammatory process.

The immune system is a strong defense system against invading foreign pathogenic microorganisms such as bacteria viruses and cancer-causing viruses, and it is essential for the healing of injured tissues. Immune cells such as macrophages remove invading infectious microorganisms. Injury to cells evokes an acute inflammatory response that releases anti-inflammatory cytokines and pro-inflammatory cytokines. Anti-inflammatory cytokines help to heal the cellular injury. If the injury is not healed, chronic inflammation is apt to ensue. This sets in motion a cascading release of pro-inflammatory cytokines that are toxic to the cells.

The results discussed in this section support the idea that increased oxidative stress and chronic inflammation play a critical role in the initiation and progression of heart disease. In the following chapter, we will examine the role of antioxidants in greater detail, given that they may be our best hope of mitigating the incidence of this crippling, complex disease.

4 The Antioxidant Defense System

History and Actions, Sources, and Properties of Antioxidants

Why are antioxidants so important, what exactly do they do for us, and how can we ensure that we are receiving enough of them to maintain optimal health and prevent the onset of disease?

First of all antioxidants have many valuable roles to play in safeguarding human health. Given that they are so successful in neutralizing free radicals, many people believe that this is their only function. However, in view of recent advances in antioxidant research, this belief has been proven to be incorrect. The actions of antioxidants on cells and tissues are varied and complex. Antioxidants work to:

1. Alter gene expression profiles
2. Alter protein kinase activity
3. Decrease markers of pro-inflammatory cytokines
4. Increase immune function
5. Induce cell differentiation (maturation) in normal cells during development
6. Participate in several biological processes
7. Prevent the release and toxicity of excessive amounts of glutamate (a key compound in cellular metabolism)

8. Scavenge free radicals

9. Activate a nuclear transcriptional factor Nrf2 by reactive oxygen species (ROS)-dependent and independent mechanisms for increasing the levels of antioxidant enzymes.

In humans the antioxidant defense system is divided into two groups: exogenous and endogenous. Exogenous antioxidants are not made in the body but rather are consumed through diet or via supplementation (standard dietary antioxidants). Endogenous antioxidants are made in the body.

Standard dietary antioxidants that are commonly consumed via the diet and used in multivitamin preparations include vitamins A, C, E, and beta-carotene. Herbal, fruit, and vegetable antioxidants include resveratrol, curcumin, cinnamon extract, and ginseng extract. B vitamins are also an essential component of an effective micronutrient preparation. Although they are not considered an antioxidant, I am including them here and in subsequent chapters and discussions because of their importance to overall health and their role in the prevention and management of heart disease.

Endogenous antioxidants include antioxidant enzymes such as superoxide dismutase (SOD); catalase and glutathione peroxidase; and compounds such as glutathione, alpha-lipoic acid, coenzyme Q10, L-carnitine, and melatonin. Antioxidant enzymes are not effective when taken orally because they are degraded in the intestinal tract. However, they can be enhanced by reactive oxygen species (ROS)-dependent and -independent activation of a nuclear transcription factor (Nrf2).

Although trace minerals of iron, copper, and manganese are essential for the activities of antioxidant enzymes and other biological activities of the body, a slight increase in the levels of free iron, copper, and manganese can amplify the production of free radicals and subsequently increase the risk of chronic disease. Therefore, it is not a good idea to add these trace minerals to a multivitamin preparation.

In this chapter* we will more fully explore the antioxidant defense system and the roles that antioxidants play in safeguarding the body's general health and well-being. We will also detail the history of antioxidants and their actions, list various sources of them, and provide other information about these very important substances.

HISTORY AND ACTIONS
OF EXOGENOUS ANTIOXIDANTS

Vitamin A

Night blindness, which we now know is caused by vitamin A deficiency, existed for centuries before the discovery of vitamin A. As early as 1500 BCE, Egyptians knew how to cure night blindness. Roman soldiers suffering from this condition traveled to Egypt where they received liver extract as treatment. (Today it is well established that liver is the richest source of vitamin A.) Treating night blindness with liver extract was not employed outside of Egypt for centuries, perhaps because medical establishments in other countries during that period did not deem it to be an acceptable treatment protocol. In 1912 Dr. Elmer McCollum of the University of Wisconsin discovered vitamin A in butter, at which time it was named fat-soluble A. The structure of vitamin A was determined in 1930, and it was synthesized in the laboratory in 1947.

In addition to playing a key role in maintaining vision, vitamin A also destroys free radicals, stimulates immune function, and regulates gene activity and embryonic development. As well it plays a role in reproduction, bone metabolism, and skin health.

B Vitamins

All of the B vitamins were discovered between 1912 and 1934. In the year 1912, the Polish biochemist Dr. Casimur Funk isolated their active substances from the rice husks of unpolished rice; these active substances

---

*Much of the material in this chapter is derived from my earlier book *Fight Diabetes with Vitamins and Antioxidants*, Rochester, Vt.: Healing Arts Press, 2014.

prevented the disease beriberi. This disease affects many parts of the body including muscle tissue, the heart, the nervous system, and the digestive tract. Dr. Funk named the substances he discovered vitamines, because he thought they were "amines" derived from ammonia. In 1920 the *e* was dropped when it became known that not all vitamins are "amines." Today there are many different vitamins in the vitamin B family.

B vitamins are essential for bodily functions such as energy production and making red blood cells. They are also helpful in the production of hormones and assisting with the maintenance of DNA.

Vitamin C

The symptoms of scurvy were known to Egyptians as early as 1500 BCE. In the fifth century, Hippocrates described its symptoms, which included bleeding gums, hemorrhaging, and death. Native American Indians had a cure for it, which involved drinking an extract made from bark and needles of the pine tree, prepared like a tea. This remedy, however, remained limited to their own population for hundreds of years. Today we know that pine bark and needles are rich in vitamin C and that scurvy is caused by a vitamin C deficiency.

During the sea voyages of European explorers between the twelfth and sixteenth centuries, the epidemic of scurvy among sailors forced some of them to land in Canada, where native Indians gave them the indigenous concoction, thereby curing their illness. In 1536 the French explorer Jacques Cartier brought this formulation to France, but the medical establishment rejected it as bogus because it had originated with the Native Americans, whom they looked down upon. In 1593 Sir Richard Hawkins began recommending that his sailors eat sour oranges and lemons to reduce the risk of disease. It would be almost another two hundred years before the British navy began recommending that ships carry sufficient lime juice for all personnel aboard. In 1928 Albert Szent-Györgyi, a Hungarian scientist, isolated hexuronic acid from the adrenal gland. This substance was vitamin C, and in 1932 it was the first vitamin to be made in the laboratory.

Vitamin C acts as an antioxidant and participates in several enzyme activities that are needed for the organs to function properly. It helps in the formation of collagen, and it also takes part in the formation of interferon, a naturally occurring anti-viral agent. In addition it regenerates damaged vitamin E to an active form of vitamin E.

Carotenoids/Beta-carotene

In 1919 carotenoid pigments were isolated from yellow plants, and in 1930 researchers found that some of the ingested carotene was converted to vitamin A. This substance is referred to as beta-carotene.

There are several types of carotenoids in plants, fruits, and vegetables. Carotenes are known to protect against ultraviolet-light-induced damage. Beta-carotene increases the expression of the connexin gene, which codes for a gap junction protein that holds two normal cells together. (Vitamin A cannot produce such an effect.) In addition, when compared to vitamin A, beta-carotene is a more effective destroyer of free radicals in an internal body environment that is marked by high oxygen pressure in the tissues.

Vitamin D

Although the bone disease rickets may have existed in human populations for centuries, it was not until 1645 that Dr. Daniel Whistler described its symptoms. In 1922 Sir Edward Mellanby discovered vitamin D while working on a cure for rickets, which vitamin D proved to be. This vitamin was later found to require sunlight for its formation in skin cells. The chemical structure of vitamin D was determined by German scientist Dr. Adolf Windaus in 1930. Vitamin D$_3$ is the most active form of vitamin D. It was chemically characterized in 1936 and was initially thought to be a steroid effective in the treatment of rickets.

In addition to being essential in bone formation, vitamin D regulates calcium and phosphorus levels in the blood. It also inhibits parathyroid hormone secretions from the parathyroid glands and stimulates immune functioning by promoting phagocytosis.

Vitamin E

In 1922 Dr. Herbert Evans of the University of California, Berkeley, observed that rats reared exclusively on whole milk grew normally but were not fertile. Fertility was restored when they were fed wheat germ. However, it took another fourteen years before the active substance that was responsible for restoring fertility was isolated from the wheat germ. When this was achieved, Dr. Evans named the substance tocopherol, from the Greek word meaning "to bear offspring," and added *ol* at the end, signifying its chemical status as an alcohol.

Vitamin E acts as an antioxidant, regulates genetic activity, and relocates certain proteins from one compartment to another within the same cell. It helps to maintain skin health, reduces scarring, and acts as an anticoagulant at very high doses. Vitamin E also reduces inflammation and stimulates immune function. Its derivative, vitamin E succinate, is considered to be the most effective form of vitamin E.

Polyphenols

Polyphenols are a very numerous group of chemical substances found in plants; they are also referred to as phytochemicals. Although plant-derived products have been used in Asia for centuries, the term polyphenol has only been in use since 1894. However, the biological actions of polyphenols and their value in human health have been clarified during the last forty years or so. Polyphenols include tannins, lignins, and flavonoids. The largest and the most widely studied polyphenols are the flavonoids, which include quercetin, epicatechin, and oligomeric proanthocyanidins.

All flavonoids possess varying degrees of antioxidant activity. They also reduce inflammation and regulate genetic activity.

ACTIONS OF ENDOGENOUS ANTIOXIDANTS

Endogenous antioxidants, as we have learned, are made in the body. They include antioxidant enzymes and compounds, some of which are detailed below.

Alpha-Lipoic Acid

Alpha-lipoic acid is a more potent antioxidant than vitamin C or vitamin E. It regenerates tissue levels of vitamin C and vitamin E and markedly elevates glutathione levels in cells. Alpha-lipoic acid participates in several enzyme activities.

Catalase

The antioxidant enzyme catalase needs iron for its biological activity; it destroys hydrogen peroxide in cells, converting it into hydrogen and water.

Coenzyme Q10

The heart and the liver, which require the most energy, have the highest concentrations of coenzyme Q10 due to the large number of mitochondria found in these organs. Other organelles inside the cells that contain coenzyme Q10 include endoplasmic reticulum, peroxisomes, lysosomes, and the Golgi apparatus.

Coenzyme Q10 is a weak antioxidant, but it is significant because it recycles vitamin E to an active form. Coenzyme Q10 is essential for generating energy within mitochondria, thereby generating energy for all of the cells of the human body.

Glutathione

Glutathione is formed in the body from three amino acids: L-cysteine, L-glutamic acid, and L-glycine. It is present in all of the cells in a reduced or oxidized form, with the highest concentration of it found in the liver. In healthy cells more than 90 percent of glutathione is present in the reduced form. The oxidized form of glutathione can be converted to the reduced form by the enzyme glutathione reductase; this reduced form acts as an antioxidant.

Glutathione is one of the most important antioxidants in that it protects cellular components inside of the cells. It is needed for the detoxification of certain exogenous toxins as well as for toxins that are produced as by-products of normal metabolism. Glutathione also participates in several enzyme activities and reduces inflammation. The antioxidant enzyme glutathione peroxidase requires selenium for its biological activity; it is responsible for removing hydrogen peroxide. This enzyme participates in the formation of glutathione.

L-carnitine

L-carnitine is synthesized from the amino acids lysine and methionine, primarily in the liver and the kidneys. It exists as L-carnitine, a biologically active form, and as D-carnitine, a biologically inactive form. Vitamin C is necessary for its synthesis. L-carnitine helps cells to break down fat and obtain energy from fat reserves. It also helps to reduce oxidative stress.

Melatonin

Melatonin is valuable in that it regulates circadian rhythms through its receptor. It also acts as an antioxidant, reduces inflammation, and stimulates immune function. Unlike other antioxidants, damaged melatonin cannot be regenerated by other antioxidants.

Superoxide Dismutase (SOD)

The antioxidant enzyme SOD requires manganese, copper, or zinc for its biological activity. Manganese (Mn)-SOD is present in the mitochondria whereas copper (Cu)-SOD and zinc (Zn)-SOD are present in the cytoplasm and the nucleus of the cell. They can destroy free radicals and hydrogen peroxide.

EXOGENOUS ANTIOXIDANTS (STANDARD DIETARY ANTIOXIDANTS) AND THEIR SOURCES

As we know vitamins A, C, and E, as well as carotenoids and the mineral selenium, are exogenous antioxidants that are also referred to as "standard dietary antioxidants," because they are commonly consumed through diet (or used in a multivitamin preparation). Other types of exogenous antioxidants include various kinds of polyphenols found in fruits, vegetables, and herbs. (Some of these polyphenols are often added to a multivitamin preparation in small quantities.)

We will discuss sources of standard dietary antioxidants next, detailing how one may obtain them from one's diet.

Vitamin A

Liver from beef, pork, chicken, turkey, and fish is the richest source of vitamin A (6.5 mg of vitamin A per 100 grams of liver). Vitamin A is also found in sweet potatoes, carrots, leafy greens, and squash, as well as in melons, peppers, tuna, and apricots.

B Vitamins

Sources of B vitamins include Brewer's yeast, cereals, milk, leafy vegetables, liver, and intestinal bacteria.

Vitamin C

The richest dietary sources of vitamin C are fruits and vegetables. They include rose hips, red peppers, parsley, guava, kiwi fruit, broccoli, lychee, papaya, and strawberries. Each of these fruits or vegetables contains approximately 2,000 mg of vitamin C per 100 grams of fruit. Other sources of vitamin C include oranges, lemons, melon, garlic, cauliflower, grapefruit, raspberries, tangerines, passion fruit, spinach, and limes. They contain about 30 to 50 mg of vitamin C per 100 grams of fruits and vegetables.

Carotenoids/Beta-carotene

The richest sources of carotenoids are sweet potatoes, carrots, spinach, mangoes, cantaloupes, apricots, kale, broccoli, parsley, cilantro, pumpkins, winter squash, and fresh thyme. However, there are more than six hundred carotenoids in various plants, fruits, and vegetables. Among them, beta-carotene, alpha-carotene, lycopene, lutein, xanthophylls, zeaxanthin, and beta-cryptoxanthin are significant. (We do not know much about many of the other carotenoids.) Beta-carotene, alpha-carotene, lycopene, and lutein have been studied extensively in laboratory experiments and in humans.

Vitamin E

The richest sources of vitamin E include wheat germ oil (215 mg per 100 of grams of oil), sunflower seed oil (56 mg per 100 grams of oil), olive oil (12 mg per 100 grams of oil), almond oil (39 mg per 100 grams of oil), hazelnut oil (26 mg per 100 grams of oil), walnut oil (20 mg per 100 grams of oil), and peanut oil (17 mg per 100 grams of oil). Sources for small amounts of vitamin E (0.1 to 2 mg per 100 grams) include kiwi fruit, fish, leafy vegetables, and whole grains. In the United States, fortified breakfast cereals are very good sources of vitamin E.

At present, most of the natural form of vitamin E is extracted from vegetable oils, primarily soybean oil. Vitamin E exists in eight different forms: four tocopherols (alpha-, beta-, gamma-, and delta-tocopherol), and four tocotrienols (alpha-, beta-, gamma-, and delta- tocotrienol). Of these alpha-tocopherol has the most biological activity. Vitamin E also exists in the natural form, commonly indicated as "d." The synthetic form is referred to as "dl." The stable esterified form of vitamin E is available as alpha-tocopheryl acetate, alpha-tocopheryl succinate, and alpha-tocopheryl nicotinate.

L-carnitine

L-carnitine is made in the body, but we can also obtain it from our diet. The highest concentration of L-carnitine is found in red meat (95 mg per 3.0 ounces of meat). In contrast chicken breast has only 3.9 mg per 3.5 ounces. L-carnitine is present in all cells of the body.

Polyphenols

As mentioned previously polyphenols are present in herbs, fruits, and vegetables. Examples of them include resveratrol (found in grape skin and seeds), curcumin (found in the spice turmeric), ginseng extract, cinnamon extract, and garlic extract. Resveratrol in particular has drawn a great deal of attention in recent years; it is found in grape skin and grape seed. As we've learned other polyphenols include tannins, lignins, and flavonoids. Major sources of flavonoids include all of the citrus fruits, berries, ginkgo biloba, onions, parsley, tea, red wine, and dark chocolate. Over five thousand naturally occurring flavonoids have been characterized from various plants.

EXOGENOUS ANTIOXIDANTS AND THEIR COMMERCIAL SOURCES

Next we will examine the commercial availability of some of the major antioxidants.

Vitamin A

Vitamin A is sold commercially as retinyl palmitate, retinyl acetate, and retinoic acid and its analogs. Retinyl acetate or retinyl palmitate (a stable form sold commercially) is converted to retinol in the intestine before absorption. Retinol is then converted to retinoic acid in the cells, where it performs all the functions of vitamin A except that of maintaining vision. Retinoic acid and its derivatives are used in laboratory studies because they're readily soluble in fat and thus enter cells easily. Vitamin A in the blood takes the form of retinol and is stored in the liver as retinyl palmitate.

Vitamin A exists as a protein-bound molecule. The vitamin A product retinoic acid is stored in all of the tissues of the body.

Alpha-Lipoic Acid

Alpha-lipoic acid is commercially available and should be added to a multivitamin preparation for the following reasons. It is a more potent antioxidant than vitamin C or vitamin E. It is soluble in both water and lipid. Therefore, it protects cellular membranes as well as water-soluble compounds. It regenerates tissue levels of vitamin C and vitamin E and markedly elevates glutathione levels in cells. Alpha-lipoic acid also participates in several enzyme activities.

B Vitamins

The B vitamins are available in the following compounds: Vitamin B_1, as thiamine mononitrate; vitamin B_2, as riboflavin; vitamin B_3, as niacinamide ascorbate; vitamin B_6, as pyridoxine hydrochloride; Folic acid, as folate; vitamin B_{12}, as cyanocobalamin; and pantothenic acid, as d-calcium pantothenate.

Vitamin C

Vitamin C is commercially sold as ascorbic acid, sodium ascorbate, magnesium ascorbate, calcium ascorbate, and timed-release capsules containing ascorbic acid and vitamin C-ester.

Vitamin C is present in all the cells of the body, and all mammals make vitamin C with the exception of guinea pigs and humans. (An adult goat makes about 13 grams of vitamin C every day.) Vitamin C can recycle the non-antioxidant form of vitamin E (the oxidized form of vitamin E) to an antioxidant form. Ascorbic acid supplements at high doses can cause an upset stomach in some people. Additionally, it should be noted that 1 gram of sodium ascorbate contains 124 mg of sodium. This form of vitamin C at high doses may thus increase the concentration of sodium in the urine, which can lead to chronic irritation of the bladder. It should also be noted that timed-release capsules of vitamin C contain additional synthetic chemicals, and that vitamin C-ester cannot function as vitamin C until the enzyme esterase removes the ester.

For these reasons we recommend calcium ascorbate. It is buffered and is unlikely to produce stomach upset or other complications.

Carotenoids/Beta-carotene

Beta-carotene is commercially available in natural or synthetic forms. Laboratory experiments have demonstrated that the natural form of beta-carotene is more effective in reducing the risk of cancer than the synthetic form. Synthetic preparations of beta-carotene also contain unknown impurities, the toxicity of which remains uncertain. Preparations of natural carotenoids primarily contain beta-carotene;

however, other types of carotenoids are also present. One molecule of beta-carotene forms two molecules of vitamin A, and 1 IU (international unit) of vitamin A equals 0.6 micrograms of beta-carotene.

Coenzyme Q10

Coenzyme Q10 is sold commercially as timed-release capsules or simply coenzyme Q10. A comparative study regarding the efficacy of timed-release and the regular forms of coenzyme Q10 has not been made. We recommend a regular form of coenzyme Q10.

Vitamin E

Vitamin E is a term used for all tocopherols and tocotrienols possessing the biological activity of alpha-tocopherol. Both tocopherol and tocotrienol have alpha (α), beta (β), gamma (γ), and delta (δ) forms. Alpha-tocopherol has the highest antioxidant activity, followed by beta-, gamma-, and delta-tocopherol. In recent years research on tocotrienols has revealed some of their valuable biological functions.

The activity of vitamin E is generally expressed in international units (IU). It is determined that 1 IU of vitamin E equals 0.66 mg of d-alpha-tocopherol, and 1 IU of racemic mixture (dl-form) equals 0.45 mg of d-alpha-tocopherol.

Vitamin E is commercially sold as d- or dl-tocopherol, alpha-tocopheryl acetate, or alpha-tocopheryl succinate (vitamin E succinate). Alpha-tocopheryl acetate and vitamin E succinate are more stable than alpha-tocopherol. Alpha-tocopherol, alpha-tocopheryl acetate, and vitamin E succinate have been widely used in laboratory and clinical studies.

Glutathione

Glutathione is sold commercially for oral consumption; however, this antioxidant is totally destroyed in the intestine. Therefore, oral administration of glutathione doesn't increase the level of glutathione in the cells and therefore will not produce any beneficial effects in the body.

Melatonin

Melatonin is a naturally occurring hormone produced primarily by the pineal gland in the brain. It is also produced by the retina, lens, and gastrointestinal tract. Melatonin is formed from the amino acid tryptophan. Melatonin is also produced by various plants such as rice.

Melatonin plays a crucial role in sleep in that it regulates circadian rhythms through its receptor. It also acts as an antioxidant, reduces inflammation, and stimulates immune function. Unlike other antioxidants, damaged melatonin cannot be regenerated by other antioxidants. It is readily available commercially as a supplement but is not recommended except for those individuals who have occasional sleep problems.

N-acetylcysteine (NAC)

N-acetylcysteine (NAC) is not made in the body, but in the laboratory from the amino acid cysteine, which is used to make glutathione in the body. NAC is not destroyed in the small intestine when consumed orally, and thus can be taken as a supplement. In the body n-acetyl is removed from NAC by the enzyme esterase, and then cysteine is used to make glutathione. Alpha-lipoic acid also increases the level of glutathione by a mechanism that is different from NAC, and it is present in all cells. This function is significant because, as we have learned, orally administered glutathione is totally destroyed in the small intestine. At high doses n-acetylcysteine binds with metals and removes them from the body; however, too much NAC may cause an imbalance in these levels in the body. I have added a proprietary amount of NAC to some of the BioArmor multivitamin formulas that I have developed and recommend, which are further articulated in the later pages of this book.

NADH

NADH is the reduced form of nicotinamide adenine dinucleotide. Like L-carnitine, nicotinamide adenine dinucleotide (NAD+) and NADH are present in all of the cells in our body. NAD+ is an oxidizing agent; therefore, it can act as a prooxidant. NADH can act as an antioxidant. NAD+ accepts electron from other molecules and is reduced to the NADH form, which can recycle oxidized vitamin E to the reduced form, which can then act as an antioxidant. NADH is essential to mitochondria for the generation of energy. Clinical studies with NADH have produced no beneficial effect; therefore it is not recommended. Instead nicotinamide (vitamin B_3), which is a precursor of NAD, is recommended.

Polyphenols

Polyphenols are important antioxidants and reduce inflammation. Certain polyphenols, such as resveratrol and curcumin, can produce some beneficial effects in certain chronic diseases; therefore, they can be added to a multiple vitamin preparation. They should also be consumed regularly through diet.

SOLUBILITY OF ANTIOXIDANTS

Lipid-soluble antioxidants include vitamin A, vitamin E, carotenoids, coenzyme Q10, and L-carnitine. These fat-soluble vitamins should be taken with meals so that they can be more readily absorbed. Water-soluble antioxidants include vitamin C and glutathione. Alpha-lipoic acid is soluble in both fat and water.

HOW TO STORE ANTIOXIDANTS

Vitamin A

Vitamin A as retinyl palmitate or retinyl acetate in solid form is stable at room temperature for a few years. The solid form of retinol, or retinoic acid, is not stable at room temperature; therefore, it should be stored at 4°C (in the refrigerator) for several months. A solution of retinoic acid is stable at 4°C, stored away from light, for several weeks.

B Vitamins

B vitamins can be stored at room temperature for at least three years.

Vitamin C

Vitamin C should not be stored in liquid form because as such it is easily destroyed within a few days. Crystal or tablet forms of vitamin C can be kept at room temperature, away from light, for a few years.

Carotenoids/Beta-carotene

Most of the commercially sold carotenoids in solid form can be stored at room temperature and away from light for a few years. They should not be stored in solution because they degrade within a few days, even if they are stored in a colder environment, away from light.

Coenzyme Q10 and NADH

These antioxidants in solid forms are stable at room temperature, away from light, for a few years. The solutions of these antioxidants are stable at 4°C, away from light, for several months.

Vitamin E

Alpha-tocopherol is relatively unstable at room temperature in comparison to alpha-tocopheryl acetate and alpha-tocopheryl succinate. Alpha-tocopherol can be stored at 4°C for several weeks, but alpha-tocopheryl acetate and alpha-tocopheryl succinate can be stored at room temperature for a few years. A solution of alpha-tocopheryl succinate is stable for several months at 4°C, if kept away from light.

Glutathione, N-acetylcysteine, and Alpha-Lipoic Acid

Solid forms of glutathione, n-acetylcysteine, and alpha-lipoic acid are stable at room temperature, away from light, for a few years. The solutions of these antioxidants are stable at 4°C, away from light, for several months.

Melatonin

The powder form of melatonin is stable at room temperature for a year or more.

Polyphenols

Polyphenols are stable and can be stored in solid form at room temperature, away from light, for a few years.

CAN ANTIOXIDANTS BE DESTROYED DURING COOKING?

Some antioxidants are destroyed during cooking, some are not, and others are partially degraded. We will explore this feature next.

Vitamin A

Of all the vitamins, vitamin A appears to be the most sensitive to heat. Routine cooking does not destroy it significantly, but slow heating for a longer period of time may reduce its potency. Canning fruits and vegetables that contain vitamin A may also diminish its potency. Prolonged cold storage may diminish it as well. The vitamin A content of fortified milk powder declines substantially after two years.

B Vitamins

B vitamins are stable when vegetables or meat are baked, steamed, or barbecued. Boiling vegetables may lose some of the B vitamin's potency.

Carotenoids/Beta-carotene

Most carotenoids, especially beta-carotene, lutein, and lycopene, are not destroyed during cooking. In fact, their bioavailability improves when they are derived from a cooked or extracted preparation (such as lycopene from tomato sauce). Thus they are more easily absorbed from the intestine.

Coenzyme Q10 and NADH

Coenzyme Q10 and NADH are partially degraded during cooking.

Vitamin E

Food processing, frying, and freezing destroy vitamin E. The vitamin E content of fortified milk powder is unaffected over a two-year period.

Glutathione, N-acetylcysteine, and Alpha-Lipoic Acid

Glutathione, n-acetylcysteine, and alpha-lipoic acid can be partially destroyed during cooking.

Polyphenols

Polyphenols are not destroyed during cooking.

CONCLUDING REMARKS

Antioxidants in our body defend against damage produced by free radicals. Some antioxidants are made in the body, and others are consumed through a healthy, well balanced diet that includes plenty of fruits and vegetables. Both dietary and endogenous antioxidants are necessary for optimal health and chronic disease prevention. Thus it is important that we determine what our individual needs for them are to ensure that we are consuming the correct and appropriate amounts necessary to keep our bodies healthy and protected from all manner of disease, including heart disease. In addition to dietary and endogenous antioxidant elevation, increasing antioxidant enzymes by activation of Nrf2 through ROS-dependent and -independent mechanisms is essential for optimally reducing oxidative stress and inflammation.

It must also be said that the biological half-lives of most micronutrients are highly variable. Therefore, the selected micronutrients should be taken twice a day to maintain a steady level of them in the body. We will be discussing specific micronutrient requirements in the latter chapters of this book.

5

The Antioxidant Defense System Further Defined

Properties, Doses, and Risks

In this chapter* we will continue our discussion of antioxidants by taking a closer look at additional properties of them, such as their absorption and retention in the human body, their doses, and our requirements for them. We will also discuss any risks that may be associated with their use. Let's start by examining how the body absorbs and retains them.

HOW MUCH OF EACH ANTIOXIDANT DO WE ABSORB AND RETAIN?

Many harmful chemicals (such as mutagens that alter genetic activity) are formed during the digestion of food. The presence of adequate amounts of antioxidants can reduce the formation of these toxic chemicals. Antioxidants may also prevent mutations, which are caused by environmental toxins, from forming in the body. It must be emphasized, however, that many of the actions of antioxidants on normal

---

*Much of the material in this chapter is derived from my book *Fight Diabetes with Vitamins and Antioxidants*, Rochester, Vt.: Healing Arts Press, 2014.

cells are not due to their antioxidative actions but rather to their role in regulating gene activity. In any event maintaining adequate amounts of micronutrients, including antioxidants in the body, is vital to optimal health and chronic disease prevention.

Only about 10 percent of ingested water-soluble or fat-soluble anti-oxidants are absorbed from the intestinal tract. It has been argued by some that 90 percent of antioxidants are therefore wasted. This argu-ment has no scientific merit, for during the digestive processes many toxic substances, including mutagens (substances that alter gene activ-ity) and carcinogens (cancer-causing substances), are formed. People who consume meat form these toxic substances more than vegetar-ians do. (The consumption of organic food does not impact upon the amounts of toxins formed during the digestion of food.) A portion of these toxins are absorbed from the gastrointestinal tract, thereby potentially increasing the risk of chronic diseases over a long period of time.

The presence of increased amounts of antioxidants in the digestive tract, even if not absorbed, markedly reduces the levels of toxins formed during digestion, and thereby may potentially decrease the adverse health effects of these toxins. Thus, the unabsorbed antioxidants still perform a very useful function in reducing the levels of mutagens and other toxins.

Let's look at specific antioxidants to see how they stack up in terms of absorbability.

Vitamin A

The highest levels of vitamin A are present in the liver, and the lowest levels in the brain.

Only about 10 to 20 percent of ingested vitamin A is absorbed from the small intestine; however, normal cells characteristically do not take up more than they need to function. Liver cells are an exception. As we have learned, ingested retinyl acetate or the retinyl palmitate form of vitamin A is converted to retinol in the intestine. Retinol is further converted to retinoic acid in the cells, yet most of the body's vitamin A is stored in the liver as retinyl palmitate.

Retinol reaches its maximum level in the blood three to six hours after the ingestion of vitamin A and drops to a normal level in about twelve hours.

Alpha-Lipoic Acid

Alpha-lipoic acid is made in the body. Ingested alpha-lipoic acid is absorbed from the small intestine and is rapidly distributed into various tissues. Its by-product, dihydrolipoic acid, also acts as an antioxidant. Both substances remove metals from the body.

B Vitamins

B vitamins are absorbed from the intestinal tract using specific transporter proteins, and vitamin B_{12} also requires an intrinsic factor for absorption.

Vitamin C

As with vitamins A and E, the highest levels of vitamin C are present in the liver, and the lowest levels in the brain.

As with vitamin A, normal cells do not take up more vitamin C than they need to function. Absorption of vitamin C from the intestine varies from 20 to 80 percent, depending upon the dose. If one consumes 200 to 500 mg of vitamin C, about 50 percent will be absorbed from the intestine. To reduce the formation of cancer-causing substances in the stomach and intestine, certain amounts of unabsorbed vitamin C may be useful. Once absorbed vitamin C is rapidly distributed throughout the body.

Vitamin C enters the blood as ascorbic acid, which can be converted to dehydroascorbic acid that can be reconverted to ascorbic acid. Vitamin C is rapidly degraded in the body.

Carotenoids/Beta-carotene

Beta-carotene is primarily stored in the eyes and fatty tissue. Other carotenoids such as lycopene accumulate in the prostate more than in other organs. Lutein accumulates in the eyes more than other organs.

Only about 10 percent of ingested beta-carotene is absorbed from the small intestine, and in humans the conversion of beta-carotene to vitamin A does not occur if the body has sufficient amounts of vitamin A. Among vegetarians who do not eat eggs or dairy products, for instance, most of the beta-carotene they consume is converted to vitamin A (retinol). Among non-vegetarians (who have sufficient stores of vitamin A), such conversion does not take place.

After a portion of ingested beta-carotene is converted to retinol (vitamin A) in the intestinal tract, the remainder is distributed in the blood and tissues of the body. About twenty other carotenoids, including by-products of a variety of ingested carotenoids, also enter the blood and tissues. The turnover (rate of degradation and excretion) of beta-carotene in the blood is slow.

Coenzyme Q10

The heart and the liver are the organs containing the highest levels of coenzyme Q10.

Coenzyme Q10 is made in the body, and its level is relatively constant unless the cells are damaged. The absorption of coenzyme Q10 from the intestinal tract varies, depending upon the preparation.

Vitamin E

Vitamin E can be taken as alpha-tocopherol, alpha-tocopheryl acetate, or alpha-tocopheryl succinate (vitamin E succinate). It has been presumed that alpha-tocopheryl acetate and vitamin E succinate are converted to alpha-tocopherol in the intestinal tract before absorption. This assumption may be true as long as the stores of alpha-tocopherol in the body are not completely full. However, if they are full, a portion of vitamin E succinate can be absorbed as vitamin E succinate. Therefore, it is not necessary that all vitamin E succinate be converted to alpha-tocopherol before absorption. Vitamin E succinate enters the cells more easily than alpha-tocopherol because of its greater solubility. In addition vitamin E succinate has some unique functions that cannot be produced by alpha-tocopherol.

Alpha-tocopherol is located primarily in the membranous structures of the cells. Vitamin E reaches its maximum level in the blood four to six hours after ingestion. The turnover of vitamin E in the blood is slow.

Glutathione and N-acetylcysteine

Glutathione is a powerful antioxidant inside of the cells, but it is very sensitive to oxidative stress. The increased production of free radicals can diminish glutathione levels in the cells. As we know glutathione cannot be taken orally because it is completely degraded in the human intestine. In order to increase the level of glutathione in the body, n-acetylcysteine (NAC), which is degraded only very little in the gut and which raises the level of glutathione in cells, is recommended.

Melatonin

Ingested melatonin is absorbed from the small intestine, but it is rapidly degraded in the body, in that it is routinely removed from the plasma in thirty-five to fifty minutes.

Polyphenols

These fat-soluble antioxidants are absorbed from the intestine without significant degradation and are then distributed throughout the tissues of the body. Flavonoids, however, are poorly absorbed by the human intestinal tract. The turnover of the phenolic compound found in polyphenols in the blood is slow. These antioxidants can be consumed through diet or supplement.

WHICH ANTIOXIDANT SUPPLEMENTS
SHOULD WE TAKE?
HOW MUCH AND HOW OFTEN?

At this time the doses of antioxidants imparting the greatest benefit to human health and maximum reduction in the incidence of chronic diseases are unknown. Nevertheless, 40 percent or more of all Americans take micronutrients on a regular basis, hoping to improve their health. In addition many people with chronic diseases take these supplements in some form, with or without their doctor's approval. Many doctors do not recommend micronutrient supplements for optimal health or chronic disease prevention and treatment.

When one talks with people who are taking micronutrients on the advice of a salesperson at a vitamin store, or are doing so after having read an article in a health care magazine or because they have watched a related report on TV, it becomes evident that their decision to take supplemental nutrients has nothing to do with scientific rationale. Furthermore, the makers of most multivitamin preparations have likewise not analyzed the science carefully enough to be able to create supplements that are composed of the right elements, administered in the correct combinations, in the proper form and dose.

For example, most of the commercially sold multiple antioxidant formulas with minerals include some combination of iron, copper, and manganese—or all three. This is despite the fact that iron, copper, and manganese—when combined with vitamin C—generate excessive amounts of free radicals in the body. In addition, in the presence of antioxidants, these minerals are more readily absorbed from the intestinal tract, which increases the body's stores of them. Increased free iron in the body has been associated with several chronic human diseases, including heart disease and diabetes. Therefore, the addition of iron, copper, or manganese to any multivitamin preparation has no scientific merit in terms of ensuring optimal health or preventing chronic disease. (In cases where a person has iron-deficiency anemia, however, a short-term iron supplement with vitamin C is essential to help with iron absorption, until such time as the anemia is cured.)

Many commercially sold multiple antioxidant preparations also contain heavy metals such as vanadium and molybdenum, which are unnecessary because sufficient amounts of these metals are obtained from a normal diet. The daily consumption of them over a long period of time can increase their stores in the body because the body has no efficient way of eliminating them. This accumulation can be toxic to brain cells.

Commercial multivitamin preparations also include inositol, methionine, and choline in varying doses (30 to 60 mg). Such doses of these nutrients serve no useful purpose, because 400 to 1,000 mg are obtained daily from the diet. Para-aminobenzoic acid (PABA) is present in some multivitamin preparations. PABA has no biological function in the body. In addition it blocks the anti-bacterial effects of sulfonamides. Therefore, patients taking sulfonamides and a multivitamin preparation containing PABA may experience a diminished effectiveness of the antibiotics.

Typically, either n-acetylcysteine (NAC) or alpha-lipoic acid is found in commercially available multivitamin preparations. These agents increase glutathione levels in the cells by different pathways. Therefore, in order to increase the level of glutathione maximally, the addition of *both* NAC and alpha-lipoic acid in a multivitamin preparation is necessary.

The addition of both beta-carotene and vitamin A to a multivitamin preparation is suggested as well, because beta-carotene not only acts as a precursor of vitamin A but also has some biological functions that vitamin A does not. Unfortunately, the beneficial effects of beta-carotene have become controversial because of flawed clinical studies that have received wide publicity. Because of this the addition of beta-carotene into multivitamin preparations has been discouraged and is generally not approved by the Institutional Review Board (IRB) responsible for human studies. Approval by the IRB is required for any study on humans.

Other carotenoids such as lycopene and lutein are also necessary for good health. However, they can be obtained from a diet that includes normal servings of tomatoes (lycopene), spinach (lutein), and paprika (xanthophylls, which includes lutein), as typically these servings provide more than adequate amounts of the nutrients and at levels much higher than those normally found in vitamin supplements. Therefore, the addition of very small amounts of lycopene and lutein to a multivitamin preparation serves no useful purpose for optimal health and/or for the prevention of chronic disease. It is also true that doses of lutein and lycopene that are higher than those commonly present in a multivitamin preparation may be needed for eye and prostate health.

Two forms of vitamin E, alpha-tocopheryl acetate (commonly used in laboratory experiments) and alpha-tocopheryl succinate, should be present in a multiple antioxidant preparation because, as we have learned, vitamin E succinate is the most effective form of vitamin E. Laboratory experiments show that alpha-tocopherol (at doses of 20 to 60 micrograms per milliliter) can increase immune function, but beta-, gamma-, and delta-forms of vitamin E at similar doses can inhibit immune function. For this reason supplementation with beta-, gamma-, or delta-tocopherol is not recommended.

Similarly, tocotrienols inhibit cholesterol synthesis. Cholesterol is necessary to maintain the normal functioning of all cells, particularly brain cells. Prolonged inhibition of cholesterol production in healthy persons with normal cholesterol levels may be harmful in young adults; therefore, tocotrienols cannot be used as supplements for optimal health in this subset of the population. In addition coenzyme Q10 formation occurs in the same pathway as cholesterol. Therefore, reduction in the level of cholesterol by tocotrienol may also cause a decrease in the level of coenzyme Q10, a necessary substance for the generation of energy in the body.

As we have mentioned earlier, the optimal form of vitamin C is calcium ascorbate because it is not acidic and does not cause upset stomach (as ascorbic acid can in some people). Therefore, one should ensure that calcium ascorbate is the form of vitamin C that's included in one's multivitamin supplement. The addition of potassium ascorbate or magnesium ascorbate to a multivitamin preparation is unnecessary.

Adequate amounts of B vitamins (two to three times the RDA value) and appropriate minerals, such as selenium, zinc, and chromium, should be included in a multivitamin preparation. Supplementation with B vitamins is necessary for reducing levels of homocysteine, a risk factor for developing heart disease. The addition of certain minerals, including selenium, is essential for maintaining optimal health because it activates the antioxidant enzyme glutathione peroxidase, which makes glutathione.

It is not possible to recommend an appropriate multiple antioxidant supplement that can be useful to everyone irrespective of age, gender, general health, and disease status. Therefore, a multiple micronutrient preparation specific to individuals and their own particular health conditions and concerns, if any, should be utilized. This issue is discussed in detail in chapter 9.

IF WE EAT A BALANCED DIET, DO WE NEED SUPPLEMENTARY ANTIOXIDANTS FOR OPTIMAL HEALTH OR CHRONIC DISEASE PREVENTION?

The answer is yes. Generally, a balanced diet is one that is low in fat and high in fiber and includes plenty of fresh fruits and vegetables. This diet may be sufficient for normal growth and development, but supplementary micronutrients, including dietary and endogenous antioxidants, are significant in maintaining optimal health and for disease prevention and treatment. One would have difficulty eating fresh fruits and vegetables daily in the amounts and at the rates that maintain ideal levels of dietary antioxidants in the blood. Furthermore, older individuals have a reduced capacity to make endogenous antioxidants. Therefore, it's important to take an appropriate preparation of micronutrients containing multiple antioxidants in addition to eating a balanced diet.

It is now known that many foods (even if grown organically) have naturally occurring toxic substances as well as protective ones. In fact,

90 percent of toxins are derived from the diet, and only about 1 percent or less are man-made—such as pesticides that are sprayed on agricultural produce. A balanced diet alone cannot get rid of naturally occurring toxins; therefore, diet alone is not sufficient to prevent chronic disease in an optimal manner.

While a balanced diet will protect against vitamin deficiency and is better than one comprising junk food, the main problem with such a diet is that the concept of it is very general, and given this its interpretation may vary markedly. One person might believe, for instance, that the daily intake of one apple, one carrot, one orange, a few fresh vegetables, a little meat, a glass of milk, and some carbohydrate constitutes a balanced diet. Other people may define a balanced diet differently, and include more or less of these same foods. Even if a balanced diet were to be sufficiently defined and standardized, the same balanced diet cannot be applied to all regions of the world, because dietary and environmental toxin levels vary markedly from one region to another. Thus, supplemental antioxidants may be necessary to add to a "balanced diet," to lower the risk of chronic disease.

As previously discussed all types of diets contain both toxic and protective substances, including those diets that are organic or "balanced." The risk of chronic illness, including heart disease and diabetes, may depend in part upon the relative consumption of protective substances versus toxic ones. Since we know very little about the relative levels of toxic and protective substances in any diet, however, we cannot know whether we are consuming higher levels of protective substances versus toxic ones. To ensure a higher intake of protective agents, one should take a daily preparation of micronutrients that contain dietary and endogenous antioxidants.

THE RISK OF TAKING MICRONUTRIENTS

The risk of taking micronutrients depends upon dose, form, frequency of ingestion, and duration of consumption, as well as whether the micronutrients are taken as a single agent or as part of a multiple micronutrient preparation. For example, when vitamin C is consumed alone at high doses, it can act as both an antioxidant and a prooxidant. It can protect the body from some forms of DNA damage caused by free radicals. It can also cause some forms of DNA damage induced by free radicals. Vitamin C in combination with other antioxidants is unlikely to produce such a dual effect, because other antioxidants will prevent the adverse effect of vitamin C on DNA.

We will examine other specific toxicities next.

Vitamin A

Liver toxicity and skin reactions have been noted after a daily oral ingestion of 50,000 IU of vitamin A when taken for a year or more. Some of these changes are reversible when the vitamin is discontinued. Liver toxicity, however, can be irreversible. Up to 5,000 IU of vitamin A, taken orally and divided into two daily doses (morning and evening), is unlikely to produce major toxic effects in a normal adult. However, higher doses of vitamin A have been associated with an increased risk of bone fracture in older individuals. Ingestion of vitamin A at doses of 10,000 IU per day can increase the risk of birth defects in pregnant women.

Because of these toxicities, the Recommended Dietary Allowances (RDA) of vitamin A for adults has been reduced from 5,000 IU to 3,000 IU per day. Pregnant women should avoid taking more than 3,000 IU of vitamin A per day. Retinoic acid and other derivatives of vitamin A should not be consumed orally for general health maintenance because of the toxic effects of these compounds at low doses.

Alpha-Lipoic Acid

Like NAC, alpha-lipoic acid is also a metal chelator (it removes heavy metals from the body). For this reason long-term consumption at high doses (300 mg or higher) may induce a deficiency of important metals. As discussed earlier this is beneficial as long as it doesn't create an imbalance in the body. For specifics on proper dosing amounts, please refer to tables 9.1–9.4 on pages 148–51 of this book.

B Vitamins

B vitamins are fairly nontoxic. However, high doses of vitamins B_6 (50 mg or more) can cause peripheral neuropathy (numbness of extremities) after long-term consumption. Fortunately this effect is reversible upon discontinuation.

Vitamin C

In most healthy people, doses of vitamin C up to 10 grams per day taken orally will not produce any toxic effects. Intravenous infusion of vitamin C at doses of 50 grams or higher has produced no significant toxic effects on blood profiles of cancer patients. In certain diseases involving iron metabolism (hemochromatosis, in which the body has very high levels of iron) or copper metabolism (Wilson's disease, in which the body has excessive amounts of copper), or exposure to high levels of manganese (Parkinson's disease-like syndrome), excessive consumption of vitamin C may be harmful because vitamin C in combination with iron, copper, or manganese, in the presence of oxygen, generates excessive amounts of free radicals.

The increased urinary excretion of oxalic acid in people taking high doses of vitamin C has been interpreted to mean that this vitamin may increase the risk of kidney stones, due to the fact that an increased excretion of oxalic acid also is found in many patients with kidney stones. These could be the results of independent biochemical reactions, however, and the two events may not necessarily be linked. There were no documented cases of an elevated incidence of kidney stones among any study group taking high doses of vitamin C in a multiple micronutrient preparation.

Stomach upset in some people occurs as a result of their ingestion of high doses of ascorbic acid. It should also be understood that 124 mg of sodium are contained in 1 gram of sodium ascorbate. As a result, at high doses, this form of vitamin C may result in an elevated sodium level in the urine, which can cause bladder irritation over time, leading to increased risk of bladder cancer.

I recommend that up to 2 grams per day of vitamin C be added to a multiple micronutrient preparation. This preparation should be taken orally twice a day; it is safe in most healthy adults.

Carotenoids/Beta-carotene

The toxicity of beta-carotene has become a controversial issue. A few studies have suggested that taking synthetic beta-carotene in a daily dose of 25 mg alone can increase the risk of some forms of heart disease among groups of people who are at a higher than average risk of developing it (such as men who are heavy tobacco smokers and those who are obese). This, however, was not an unexpected result because typically the body of a heavy smoker is one that features a high oxidative environment in which beta-carotene will be oxidized, thereby acting as a prooxidant rather than as an antioxidant. There are no studies that show that if beta-carotene is present in a multiple antioxidant preparation, it will increase the risk of developing heart disease among high-risk populations.

There is no known toxicity of beta-carotene up to doses of 15 mg per day in normal persons or high-risk populations. Bronzing of the skin may appear after the oral ingestion of beta-carotene at a dose of 100 mg per day or higher, taken for over a few months. As well deposits of beta-carotene pigment may be found in the eye after the long-term consumption of high doses of beta-carotene. These excessive pigment deposits can harm the eye; however, these changes are reversible upon discontinuation of the supplement. Other carotenoids such as lutein and lycopene are nontoxic at oral doses of up to 25 mg per day.

Coenzyme Q10

Oral doses of up to 300 mg of coenzyme Q10 have been given to patients with breast cancer, and up to 1,200 mg to patients with Parkinson's disease without significant, apparent toxicity. High doses of coenzyme

Q10 have been used in the treatment of advanced heart disease without adverse effects. Doses of up to 200 mg in a multivitamin preparation taken orally every day are considered safe for most adults.

Vitamin E

In a large human trial that enrolled nine thousand healthy adults, a daily oral intake of 3,000 IU of alpha-tocopherol acetate for eleven years did not produce any major, detectable side effects, although isolated cases of fatigue, skin reactions, and upset stomach have been reported after the ingestion of high doses (higher than 1,000 IU per day) of vitamin E for a prolonged period of time. High doses of vitamin E (2,000 IU per day) can cause a blood-clotting defect, which is reversible with the administration of vitamin K. Laboratory experiments have shown that the solvents of some water-soluble preparations of vitamin E are toxic and should be avoided.

According to many studies, up to 400 IU of vitamin E per day administered in a multivitamin preparation is safe in most healthy adults. However, the same dose of vitamin E alone, if taken orally, may increase the risk of some forms of heart disease in high-risk populations (heavy tobacco smokers or those persons with a previous history of heart disease, for instance). This is due to the fact that the bodies of individuals who are at an elevated risk for heart disease have high oxidative environments in which vitamin E may be oxidized to act as a prooxidant rather than an antioxidant.

Glutathione

Glutathione is considered nontoxic at doses commonly utilized; however, and again, it cannot be absorbed when ingested orally because it is totally degraded in the intestinal tract.

N-acetylcysteine (NAC)

Doses of up to 300 to 400 mg of n-acetylcysteine in a multivitamin preparation are considered safe. High doses of NAC can bind with heavy metals such as lead and mercury and remove them from the body. However, if such doses are taken on a regular basis, they can increase the excretion of valuable minerals such as zinc, which may prove harmful.

Polyphenols

Although polyphenols have no known toxicity at doses used in several laboratory and human studies, the adverse health effects of high doses of these compounds have not been evaluated in humans. Resveratrol and curcumin at doses of 50 to 500 mg are considered safe and commonly used in multiple vitamin preparations.

Selenium and Zinc

An antioxidant enzyme, glutathione peroxidase, requires selenium in order to exert its antioxidant action. Selenium in combination with vitamin E is more effective than either micronutrient taken alone. Certain metals such as lead, cadmium, arsenic, mercury, and silver block the action of selenium.

Commercial preparations of selenium include inorganic selenium (sodium selenite) and various forms of organic selenium. Some studies have reported that sodium selenite is not absorbed adequately, whereas organic selenium, including yeast-selenium and seleno-L-methionine, is absorbed very well. For this reason seleno-L-methionine is the form of selenium most commonly used in multivitamin preparations.

The optimal doses of selenium in terms of its health benefits are unknown. In the United States, the average dietary intake of selenium is about 125 to 150 micrograms per day. The Recommended Dietary Allowances (RDA) value of selenium for adults is 55 to 70 micrograms per day. If an average person consumes 125 to 150 micrograms of selenium each day, a supplement of 100 micrograms of selenium in a multivitamin preparation is safe. High doses of selenium (400 micrograms or higher), if ingested every day for a long period of time, may induce dry skin and cataract formation in some individuals.

It is commonly believed that high doses of zinc are helpful in maintaining good health, but this may not be true. Several laboratory experiments have shown that high doses of zinc block the action of selenium. Furthermore, high doses of zinc can damage mitochondrial function, which can increase the production of free radicals. Therefore, doses higher than 15 to 25 mg of zinc in a multivitamin preparation should be avoided.

VITAMIN CONSUMPTION, COST, AND ADVERSE EFFECTS

In 2007 sales of dietary supplements reached 23.7 billion dollars, and in 2009 it was estimated that more than 50 percent of adults in the United States consumed some form of dietary supplement (National Health Interview Survey). Despite the reporting of inconsistent and occasionally negative results obtained from some flawed clinical studies in which a single antioxidant was used in a population that was at high risk for developing heart disease, the overall rate of consumption of dietary supplements has not declined.

The number of dietary supplements in the marketplace rose from approximately 4,000 in 1995 to approximately 75,000 in 2008. In addition food products such as fortified cereals and energy drinks containing a variety of dietary supplements became widely available to consumers in unprecedented numbers in these years.

In 2007 the Government Accountability Office (GAO) mandated that all adverse health events caused by the consumption of dietary supplements be reported. In 2008 the numbers reflect a 3-fold increase in the number of all adverse health events compared with 2007. The United States Food and Drug Administration (FDA) estimates that currently the total number of adverse health events that are related to the consumption of dietary supplements is more than 50,000 per year.

These adverse health events are primarily associated with the consumption of certain herbs, such as Ephedra for instance, which is considered a dietary supplement. Other types of dietary supplements such as vitamins A, C, and E, and carotenoids, glutathione, R-alpha-lipoic aid, coenzyme Q10, and L-carnitine have not produced any adverse health events for decades. However, the reported adverse health effects of certain herbs were perceived by most consumers to include the above-referenced antioxidants. I strongly believe that the reporting of any adverse health effects of certain herbs should be specific to those herbs and not extended erroneously to include other dietary supplements such as valuable antioxidants.

Similarly, the reporting of adverse effects obtained from the use of a single antioxidant such as beta-carotene in populations at high risk of developing heart disease should not lead to the assumption that taking beta-carotene in a multiple antioxidant preparation will produce results similar to those produced by beta-carotene alone. In addition the results obtained from populations at high risk of developing heart disease or diabetes should not be extrapolated to pertain to healthy adults. Unfortunately, most reports published through the media state that antioxidants can increase the risk of heart disease in populations that are at high risk for its development.

This erroneous reporting of scientific observations creates uncertainty and anxiety in the minds of those who are taking or recommending dietary supplements. In my opinion daily consumption of a micronutrient preparation containing multiple dietary and endogenous antioxidants, together with constructive changes in diet and lifestyle, may have very significant positive impacts in the maintenance of good health and the prevention of chronic diseases such as heart disease.

CONCLUDING REMARKS

Most antioxidants at certain doses are considered safe; however, some antioxidants such as vitamin A, beta-carotene, and vitamin E at high doses can be harmful after long-term daily consumption. Additionally, the window of safety for selenium and vitamin A is very narrow.

Recommended Dietary Allowances (RDA), now referred to as DRI (Daily Recommended Intakes), have been established for each micronutrient. These values are considered sufficient for preventing deficiencies and for allowing for normal growth and development. However, these values may not be sufficient for optimal health and chronic disease prevention or treatment. Furthermore, most standard antioxidants may not be obtainable in adequate amounts from one's diet alone.

Thus we believe that moderate supplementation with multiple micronutrients, including dietary and endogenous antioxidants together with a balanced diet and changes in lifestyle, are needed for optimal health and chronic disease prevention and treatment. The dosage and type of micronutrients needed depend upon a person's age, gender, prevailing medical conditions or illnesses, disease risk levels (low risk or high risk), and disease stage (early or advanced stage). These topics are addressed in chapter 9 of this book.

I recommend that daily supplementation with a micronutrient preparation containing dietary and endogenous antioxidants, B vitamins, vitamin D, and the mineral selenium (but not iron, copper, or manganese) should be employed to prevent chronic diseases such as heart disease and diabetes. Before we discuss specific recommendations, however, let's examine some of the laboratory and clinical studies that have been done using antioxidants to date.

6 The Search for Prevention

The Laboratory and Epidemiologic Studies

In spite of the current recommendations by the American Heart Association and the prevalence of early detection methods and technologies, it's an all too startling fact that heart disease is the primary cause of death in the United States. It's difficult to pinpoint exactly why this remains the case, although as stated in the preface to this book, it may be due to the fact that current mitigation strategies only target one aspect of the disease at a time, to the exclusion of other precipitating factors. Specifically, perhaps it is the case that chronic inflammation, the increased production of free radicals, and elevated levels of homocysteine are not being reduced simultaneously by current approaches to prevention.

Let's explore the application of statins for instance, as it pertains to this point. Statins are drugs that are used to reduce the development of heart disease and heart attacks in high-risk populations, and while they've proved useful in this, they've had much less of an impact on reducing oxidative stress and chronic inflammation. In addition they do not affect homocysteine levels or its mechanism of action, which is mediated by free radicals. If we were to employ a therapeutic strategy that targeted these three end points simultaneously, we might be much more successful in our overall aim of reducing the prevalence of heart disease. Specifically, if we were to use antioxidants, which neutralize free radicals and reduce chronic inflammation, together with B vitamins, which reduce homocysteine levels, we might reduce these individual risk factors simultaneously across the board, and thereby may reduce the overall incidence of heart disease in a way that current treatment options do not.

Additionally, changes in diet and lifestyle may enhance the aforementioned targeted supplementation. Currently, cardiologists and primary care doctors recommend changes in the diet and lifestyle for the prevention of heart disease, but they do not routinely recommend vitamins and antioxidant supplements for it. They fear that taking antioxidants may reduce the effectiveness of their therapy. This fear is not justified, because there is no conclusive data to support that an appropriate preparation of multiple micronutrients containing dietary and endogenous antioxidants can interfere with the efficacy of currently prescribed heart medications.

In taking a closer look at the potentially preventive and therapeutic effects of supplements on the incidence and prevalence of heart disease, we will next turn our focus to studies that have been done on this topic. These encompass laboratory experiments with animals as well as human studies that have been performed utilizing both epidemiologic studies (survey-types of studies) and clinical intervention studies.

In this chapter we will examine some of the laboratory and epidemiologic studies that have been done. In the next chapter we will continue our discussion by examining the results of clinical intervention studies in order to determine the effectiveness of micronutrients in combating heart disease. First let's review what we have learned to date.

THE EFFECTIVENESS OF ANTIOXIDANTS
IN REDUCING THE RISK OF HEART DISEASE

As we know there are several external and internal risk factors that increase one's chances of developing heart disease. Some risk factors, such as age, gender, ethnicity, and family history cannot be changed or improved upon.

Other risk factors can be changed. They include elevated oxidative stress and inflammation, obesity, physical inactivity, high blood pressure, high levels of low-density lipoprotein (LDL) cholesterol, low levels of high-density lipoprotein (HDL) cholesterol, the smoking of tobacco, and elevated levels of homocysteine and C-reactive proteins (CRP).

These risk factors individually or in combination enhance one's chances of developing heart disease by generating excessive amounts of free radicals and by causing inflammation. Sources of inflammation include infectious agents such as bacteria and viruses and damaged endothelial cells of blood vessels supplying blood to the heart.

Because increased oxidative stress and inflammation play a key role in the development of heart disease, it is possible to devise a strategy that reduces these two causative agents. Antioxidants reduce oxidative stress by destroying free radicals, and they reduce inflammation by decreasing the levels of pro-inflammatory cytokines in the body. Antioxidants also increase the levels of antioxidant enzymes by activating Nrf2 through reactive oxygen species (ROS)-dependent and -independent mechanisms. Antioxidants are naturally occurring and safe. Therefore, they should be useful in the prevention of heart disease. Indeed, the U.S. Prevention Service Task Force recommends antioxidant-containing multivitamin supplements to reduce the risk of heart disease (USPST Force 2003; Riley and Stouffer 2002).

However, these recommendations do not provide guidelines with respect to the *types* of vitamins, antioxidants, and minerals that should be included in a multivitamin preparation and those that should be excluded. Doses and dose-schedule are also not included in the recommendations. These issues will be discussed in detail in chapter 9.

Let's now turn our attention to the studies, both laboratory and epidemiologic, which have been done to date as regards heart disease.

LABORATORY STUDIES

Extensive laboratory studies using cell cultures (cells grown in petri dishes) and animals (rats, mice, and rabbits) have been utilized in the study of cardiac issues. They show the potential benefit of vitamins and antioxidants in reducing its risk. There are two kinds of laboratory studies used in this context: cell-culture studies and animal studies. Some of these studies are described next.

Cell-Culture Studies (In Vitro Studies)

Cell-culture studies are also referred to as in vitro studies. In these types of studies, rodent or human cells are grown in petri dishes and one or more antioxidants are added directly into the dishes. The effects of antioxidants on biochemical heart disease risk factors, such as markers of oxidative stress and inflammation, are determined a few days later. The results from cell-culture studies can reveal the potential value of one or more antioxidants in reducing heart disease–related biochemical risk factors. The toxicity of antioxidants can also be determined by the results of a cell-culture study.

Cell-culture studies are very useful because the experiments are performed easily and are inexpensive compared to animal or human studies. Furthermore, results can be obtained within a few days or a few weeks. These types of studies can also provide ideas on how antioxidants work on cellular and molecular levels. Many revolutionary studies have been performed using cell-culture systems. However, this type of study does have some limitations. For example, the beneficial effects of antioxidants observed in cell culture cannot predict whether or not the same effects will be observed in animals and humans. Nor are the dose and dose-schedule used in cell-culture studies applicable to the design of animal and human studies. In addition this experimental system cannot be used to determine the effects of antioxidants and vitamins on actual heart disease.

Specifically, as regards antioxidants, some cell-culture experiments have demonstrated their value in reducing the risk factors of developing heart disease. For example, vitamin E (alpha-tocopherol), and tocotrienol (a form of vitamin E that is derived from plants), prevented chemical-induced platelet aggregation (Freedman et al. 1996; Qureshi et al. 2011). Increased platelet aggregation is one of the risk factors that increase one's chances of developing certain types of heart disease. Thus, cell-culture studies support the value of a single antioxidant (vitamin E) in reducing the potential risk of heart disease. (Human studies have produced inconsistent results.)

Animal Studies (In Vivo Studies)

The other kind of laboratory studies used in evaluating the value of antioxidants in reducing the risk of heart disease are animal studies, or in vivo studies. In these studies the effects of antioxidants on chemical-induced or diet-induced heart disease, as well as levels of markers of oxidative damage and inflammation, are determined.

It is now customary to perform animal studies after in vitro studies; however, animal studies with antioxidants were historically performed long before the techniques of cell culture became readily available in the early 1960s. Animal studies are considered to be essential prior to the testing of antioxidants in humans is done, although some scientists believe that the extensive use of animals in antioxidant research is not warranted,* and that most information pertaining to beneficial or toxic effects can be obtained from normal human cell-culture studies instead. Animal studies are relatively simple and inexpensive compared to human studies. In addition the results of animal studies can be obtained within a few months rather than several years.

---

*Rats, mice, and occasionally rabbits are used to evaluate the effectiveness, as well as the toxicity, of antioxidants and vitamins in reducing the risk of heart disease.

In any event it should be remembered that animal studies with anti-oxidants provide only suggestions and potential guidance with respect to the effectiveness of antioxidants in reducing the risk of heart disease. The effective dose, dose-schedule, safety, and period of observation used in animal experiments with antioxidants cannot be utilized directly in the experimental design of human studies. This is due to the fact that the effectiveness, absorption, metabolism (turnover), excretion (elimination), and toxicity of antioxidants in animals is totally different from that of humans. In addition most mammals except for guinea pigs make their own vitamin C. Humans do not; we consume vitamin C from the diet. The presence of vitamin C in most animals can influence the effectiveness of antioxidant supplementation in reducing the risk of heart disease.

Most animal studies have utilized a single antioxidant to evaluate the effectiveness of antioxidants in reducing the development of heart disease. This is due to the fact that results can easily be explained on the basis of how the individual antioxidant actually acts in the body. It must be kept in mind that the results obtained from the use of a single antioxidant should not be correlated to the effectiveness of a vitamin preparation containing multiple antioxidants. Generally, multiple anti-oxidants are more effective than a single antioxidant. The rationale for this is discussed in chapter 8.

Animal Studies Using One or Two Antioxidants

A few selected studies on the effectiveness of one or two antioxidants in reducing the risk of heart disease in animals are described here.

Animal studies have consistently shown that supplementation with an individual antioxidant alone reduced the incidence of chemical- or diet-induced heart disease. Individual antioxidants reduced the development of different forms of heart disease by reducing oxidative stress and elevating antioxidant enzymes. These individual antioxidants utilized are as follows: vitamin E (Verlangieri and Bush 1992), alpha-lipoic acid (He et al. 2012), n-acetylcysteine (NAC) (Niwano et al. 2011), lycopene (Bohm 2012), coenzyme Q10 (Littarru et al. 2011), resvera-trol (Movahed et al. 2012), melatonin (Reiter et al. 2010), flavonols (Perez-Vizcaino and Duarte 2010), garlic (Reinhart et al. 2008), and epigallocatechin-gallate (a product derived from garlic, which has anti-oxidant activity) (Devika and Stanely Mainzen Prince 2008). However, these observations with a single antioxidant were not confirmed in some human studies. Reasons for this different response (to a single antioxi-dant) in humans and animals are discussed in chapter 8.

In some animal studies, a combination of two antioxidants (versus a single antioxidant), was used to evaluate effectiveness in reducing the risk of heart disease. It has been reported that a combination of vitamin E (alpha-tocopherol) and quercetin (a type of polyphenol) was more effective in protecting against chemical-induced myocardial infarction (heart attack) in rats than was an individual antioxidant (Punithavathi and Stanely Mainzen Prince 2011).

Excessive amounts of cholesterol increase oxidative stress in the heart and cause damage to heart muscle. A combination of vitamins E and C reduced the damaging effect of excessive amounts of cholesterol (Joseph et al. 2008). The beneficial effects of one or two dietary antiox-idants on heart disease have not been consistently observed in patients with a high risk of developing heart disease.

In summary laboratory studies (animal and cell-culture studies) have consistently shown that supplementation with a single antioxidant reduced the chemical-induced risk of heart disease. There were no harmful effects of any antioxidant tested in these studies.

HUMAN EPIDEMIOLOGIC STUDIES

Human studies are very costly and time-consuming, but they are essen-tial in demonstrating the value of vitamins and antioxidants in reduc-ing the risk of developing heart disease. Human studies are performed in two different ways. One way is to perform an epidemiologic study (survey-type study); the other way is to perform an intervention study wherein one group of patients receives an oral supplementation of vitamins and the other group of patients receives placebo pills, which don't contain vitamins, in a similar manner.

Epidemiologic studies are time and labor intensive, but less expensive and easier to perform than intervention studies. However, epidemiologic studies can only establish an *association* between an intake of vitamins and antioxidants from the diet, and the risk of developing heart disease.

Only intervention studies can provide conclusive proof about the effectiveness of vitamins and antioxidants in this particular line of research. Two kinds of epidemiologic studies have been used in this regard: retrospective case-control studies and prospective case-control studies. Let's look at these studies next.

The Retrospective Case-Control Study

In a *retrospective case-control study*, a set of questions is provided to patients; these questions pertain to their past history (activities of the last week, the last month, the last year, and so on) as to dietary patterns and/or vitamin supplements. Questions about gender, age, weight, lifestyle (smoking habits, stress levels, physical activity, and so on). From the answers obtained on the diet and vitamin-supplement intake questionnaire, the patients' consumption of vitamins, antioxidants, fats, and fiber is estimated, using appropriate nutritional computer software.

The patients are divided into at least two major groups; age and gender are generally matched between them. One group has the highest intake of antioxidants from the diet or from supplements. The other group has the lowest intake of antioxidants from the diet or from supplements. The risk of developing heart disease is then compared between the two groups. From this comparison the association between dietary intake of vitamins or vitamin supplements and heart disease is established. The association could be that an intake of vitamins from the diet or from vitamin supplements reduced the risk of developing heart disease or that it had no effects or that it had harmful effects.

Generally, in epidemiologic studies, the dietary patterns and vitamin supplementation with respect to the type, dose, dose-schedule, and number of vitamins differ markedly from one individual to another. Therefore, it is difficult to make an association between those with an increased intake of antioxidants from the diet or vitamin supplements and a reduced risk of developing heart disease.

The Prospective Case-Control Study

In a *prospective case-control study,* a set of questions regarding one's diet, vitamin supplements, gender, age, weight, lifestyle (smoking habits, stress levels, physical activity, and so on), is provided to the individuals participating in the study in order to establish baseline information *before* the start of the experiment. The participating individuals are given a record book with the aforementioned set of questions and asked to keep a record of the food they consume and the vitamin supplements they take each and every day.

At the end of a period of years (typically five to ten years), the intake of vitamins, fat, and fiber from the dietary records of participating individuals is estimated, using appropriate nutritional computer software. The risk of heart disease between those who had a higher intake of vitamins and those who had a lower intake of vitamins is then compared. The association could be that a higher intake of vitamins reduced the development of heart disease or it had no effects or it had harmful effects.

Generally, in this type of epidemiologic study, the dietary patterns and vitamin supplements with respect to the type, dose, dose-schedule, and number of vitamins differ markedly from one individual to another. Therefore, as with the retrospective case-control study, it's difficult to make an association between those with an increased intake of antioxidants from the diet or vitamin supplements and a reduced risk of developing heart disease. This type of survey, however, remains more useful than the retrospective case-control study, because the information about one's diet, supplements, and lifestyle is obtained from a record book written daily during the course of the experiment rather than being based on one's memory, which may be faulty.

In any case the results (positive or negative) of epidemiologic studies alone cannot be used to develop public policy for recommending vitamin supplements for reducing the risk of heart disease.

As we know, in most survey-types of studies, the daily intake of antioxidants such as vitamin A, vitamin C, vitamin E, beta-carotene, and B vitamins is determined from answers given on dietary questionnaires or records. Occasionally, the blood levels of antioxidants are determined. The association between a daily intake of individual antioxidants and the blood levels of individual antioxidants, and the risk of developing heart disease is determined. A review of nine previously published survey-type studies involving 293,172 individuals with a follow-up period of ten years showed that a high intake of dietary vitamin C, but not vitamin E or carotenoids, was associated with a reduced risk of heart disease (Knekt et al. 2004).

The European Cancer-Norfolk Population-Based Study recruited 20,926 men and women ages forty to seventy-nine to evaluate the role of plasma levels of vitamin C in maintaining blood pressure. The vitamin C was derived from the consumption of dietary fruits and vegetables. The results showed that the blood pressure of individuals with the highest levels of plasma vitamin C was 22 percent lower compared to those who had the lowest levels of plasma vitamin C (Myint et al. 2011).

Using the same population and the same experimental setup involving 9,187 apparently healthy men and 11,112 apparently healthy women, it was demonstrated that elevated plasma levels of vitamin C were associated with a reduction in the risk of heart failure (Pfister et al. 2011).

In the Japan Collaborative Cohort Study (JACC) involving 23,119 men and 35,611 women ages forty to seventy-nine without a previous history of heart disease, the association between a dietary intake of vitamin A, vitamin C, vitamin E, and mortality from heart disease was determined. The results showed that an increased intake of vitamin C from fruits and vegetables was associated with a reduction in mortality from heart disease in both men and women. No significant association was found between an intake of vitamin A or vitamin E and the risk of dying from heart disease (Kubota et al. 2011).

Increased carotid artery intima media thickness (IMT; the thickness of the wall of the carotid artery) may elevate the risk of atherosclerosis and heart disease. Increased IMT leads to a narrowing of the coronary artery, which can cause a reduced blood supply to the heart. In a survey-type of study in Finland involving 1,212 men ages sixty-one to eighty, the association between plasma levels of carotenoids and coronary IMT was determined. The results showed that high plasma concentrations of beta-cryptoxanthin, lycopene, and alpha-carotene were associated with a reduction in coronary IMT (Karppi et al. 2011).

In the Singapore Chinese Health Study, which involved 63,257 Chinese men and women ages forty-five to seventy-four, the association between plasma levels of vitamin A (retinol) or carotenoids and the risk of developing acute myocardial infarction was determined. The results showed that among the carotenoids, only elevated plasma levels of beta-cryptoxanthin and lutein were associated with a decreased risk of heart attack (Koh et al. 2011).

A review of twelve epidemiologic studies showed that an increased intake of vitamin E or vitamin A from the diet was associated with a reduction in mortality from heart disease (Gey and Puska 1989).

In a Polish study, lower levels of plasma vitamin E were associated with stable and unstable angina (Sklodowska 1991).

In a study done in the United Kingdom, lower levels of plasma vitamin E were associated with an increased risk of angina (Riemersma et al. 1991).

In a Harvard study of 39,910 male health professionals, a 36 percent lower relative risk of heart disease was demonstrated among those consuming 60 IU of vitamin E per day in comparison to those consuming fewer than 7.5 IU of vitamin E per day (Rimm et al. 1993). Men who took at least 100 IU of vitamin E per day for at least two years had a 37 percent lower risk of heart disease than those who did not take this vitamin.

Another Harvard study of 87,245 healthy nurses with a follow-up period of eight years revealed that women with the highest vitamin E intake had a 34 percent lower relative risk of major cardiac events in comparison to those with the lowest levels of vitamin E (Stampfer et al. 1993). The relative risk of heart disease was 48 percent lower in women taking vitamin E supplements (higher than 100 mg per day), for at least two years.

An intake of vitamin E obtained only from the diet provided no such protection against heart disease.

The results of several studies on the use of dietary or supplemental antioxidants suggest that an increased intake of vegetables, nuts, and other staples of the Mediterranean diet is associated with a decreased risk of heart disease (Mente et al. 2009). To a lesser extent, similar findings were noted with an increased intake of fish, marine omega-3 fatty acids, folate, whole grains, dietary vitamins C, E, and beta-carotene, and any kind of alcohol, fruit, and fiber. These studies reveal that changes in diet, together with vitamin supplements, may be very valuable in reducing the risk of heart disease.

In an Italian study involving 29,689 women, the value of consuming leafy vegetables, olive oil, and fruit was tested (Bendinelli et al. 2011). The results showed that the women who ate the highest amounts of leafy vegetables and olive oil had a reduced risk of heart disease; however, consuming fruits alone had no effect on the risk of developing heart disease.

No epidemiologic studies have evaluated the effectiveness of the intake of combined vitamin A, beta-carotene, vitamin C, vitamin E, selenium, and B vitamins in reducing the risk of heart disease. None of the epidemiologic studies have examined the role of endogenous antioxidants such as glutathione, alpha-lipoic acid, L-carnitine, or coenzyme Q10 in reducing the risk of heart disease. This could be due to the fact that such a study would require a determination of plasma levels of endogenous antioxidants, which is logistically problematic given that it is difficult to (a) collect the participants' blood and (b) determine the endogenous levels in it (in the laboratory). Techniques for so doing are not readily available to most epidemiologists.

Given the experimental designs of the aforementioned epidemiologic studies, which have several inherent technical issues, it is difficult to arrive at any definitive conclusions with respect to the value of antioxidants in reducing the risk of heart disease. These inherent technical problems include the following:

(a) The collection of retrospective dietary history data via questionnaires is unreliable because it's based on the memories of the study participants. Quantitative and qualitative information on past daily dietary intake of vitamins and antioxidants are impossible to recall with a high degree of accuracy.

(b) An intake of antioxidants or B vitamins from the dietary records is difficult to express in a quantitative manner because the information on antioxidant intake is based on estimations of the types of food consumed and their approximate quantities rather than actual measurements. Thus, a determination of the dietary intake of antioxidants, B vitamins, fat, and fiber on the basis of a dietary history or a dietary record must be considered unreliable until such time that these intake amounts may be validated by blood level measurements of these nutrients.

What is true of epidemiologic studies is that, in addition to dietary issues, there are several other confounding factors associated with lifestyle and the environment that may impact the risk of heart disease. It is very difficult to match the factors of diet, lifestyle, and the environment of the group with a high intake of antioxidants from the diet or from supplements, with the same variables in a second group having a lower intake of antioxidants. In other words, if all of these variables were equal between both groups, it would be a much easier matter to measure how the intake of dietary or supplemental antioxidants impacts the risk of developing heart disease.

It should also be emphasized that epidemiologic studies, even those having a strong experimental design and correct data interpretation, can only *infer* a beneficial or harmful relationship between single or multiple antioxidants and the risk of heart disease. The cause-effect relationship between vitamin intake and the risk of heart disease can only be definitively established by a well-designed intervention trial in high-risk human populations.

CONCLUDING REMARKS

In this chapter we have examined some different types of studies in order to determine the value of antioxidants on heart disease. In summary laboratory studies (animal and cell-culture studies) have consistently shown that supplementation with a single antioxidant reduced the chemical-induced risk of heart disease. There were no harmful effects of any antioxidant tested in these studies. Almost all of the epidemiologic studies revealed the possibility that an increased intake of antioxidants from the diet and/or supplements could be beneficial in preventing heart disease. These studies primarily focused on establishing an association between an increased intake of vitamin E alone and a reduction in the risk of heart disease. One of the end results was that no harmful association between an intake of single antioxidants and the risk of heart disease was observed. In addition increased consumption of leafy vegetables and olive oil was associated with a decreased risk of heart disease.

These studies have outlined a clear path ahead, but again we must ask: Why does it remain the case that heart disease is the number one cause of death in the United States, with stroke clocking in at number four? In this author's view, this is due in large measure to the fact that current strategies do not target three primary end goals at the same time. Chronic inflammation, the increased production of free radicals, and elevated levels of homocysteine are not being reduced simultaneously by current approaches to prevention. Perhaps if a three-pronged strategy to address these factors were employed and employed consistently, we might see a reduction in the number of strokes and deaths from heart disease.

Also, currently cardiologists and primary care doctors recommend changes in one's diet and lifestyle for the prevention of heart disease, but they do not routinely recommend vitamins and antioxidant supplements for same. Furthermore, if people do take supplements in the hopes of improving their health or curing their condition or illness, they typically do so based on hearsay or with a layperson's relatively uneducated understanding. Coupled with this is the fact that supplements available on the market today have not been designed based on a thorough scientific analysis of how these substances act and interact in the human body. There is much to be gained from a productive exploration of the value of vitamins and antioxidants from a firm scientific perspective, as I hope is clear from the views I have articulated in the pages of this book.

In the following chapter we will examine the human intervention studies that have been conducted to date, to see how their results may shed light on and provide further insights on the matter at hand.

7

The Search for Prevention Further Defined

The Intervention Studies

The laboratory and human epidemiologic studies discussed in the previous chapter showed the possibility of beneficial effects of some individual dietary antioxidants in reducing the risk of heart disease. This made it essential to test the effectiveness of supplemented antioxidants in reducing the risk of heart disease in humans.

We will discuss the results of some of these clinical intervention studies in this chapter. Before doing that, however, let's take a look at the design of a typical intervention study with micronutrient supplements and examine some factors to consider when constructing one.

COMMON CONCERNS ASSOCIATED WITH THE DESIGN OF A TYPICAL INTERVENTION STUDY

In order to perform a meaningful clinical study in which patients are given oral doses of vitamin supplements daily, the following points must be considered:

1. What are the appropriate patient populations for the study of heart disease?
2. What are the blood levels of the markers of oxidative stress and chronic inflammation in patients selected for the study?
3. How many vitamins and antioxidants (single vs. multiple) should be used in the proposed study?
4. What form, type, dose, and dose-schedule of vitamins and anti-oxidants should be used in the proposed study?
5. What type of the primary and secondary end points (clinical outcomes) should be measured at the end of the study?
6. How long should the study period be in order that it yields meaningful results?

Let's look at these concerns in more detail below, specifically as these criteria pertain to the study of heart disease.

What are the appropriate patient populations? For a heart disease prevention study, the population selected for study should be one that is at a high risk for developing heart disease. High-risk populations commonly used in these clinical intervention studies include heavy tobacco smokers, older individuals (ages fifty to seventy), individuals with a family history of heart disease, obese individuals, and patients with type 2 diabetes. The main reason for selecting a high-risk population is that, with them, the effectiveness of vitamin supplements on the risk of heart disease can be determined within a shorter period of time.

What are the blood levels of the markers of oxidative stress and chronic inflammation in patients selected for the study? High-risk populations for developing heart disease have high blood levels of markers of oxidative stress and inflammation. This provides an opportunity to evaluate the effectiveness of vitamin supplements in reducing these markers. In published studies on antioxidants and heart disease, the types of populations have markedly varied from one clinical study to another. As much as possible, this should be standardized in future studies because it is one of the reasons for the inconsistent results that have contributed to the ongoing confusion about the value of antioxidants in reducing the risk of heart disease.

How many vitamins and antioxidants (single vs. multiple) should be used in the proposed study? This is a very important question and one that has been ignored in most clinical studies. Although laboratory and human epidemiologic studies showed that single antioxidants could be useful in reducing the risk of heart disease, the use of individual antioxidants in high-risk populations may produce transient benefits, no effects, or even harmful effects. This is due to the fact that a single antioxidant such as vitamin E or beta-carotene, when administered to an individual who has a high internal oxidative environment, would be oxidized and would then act as a prooxidant (a free radical) rather than as an antioxidant. The continued presence of increased amounts of the prooxidant form of an antioxidant would be ineffective after a short period of antioxidant treatment or it would increase the risk of developing heart disease in high-risk populations after long-term consumption. If the same oxidant is present in a multivitamin preparation, the presence of other antioxidants would prevent the conversion of the administered antioxidant to a prooxidant. Therefore, taking individual vitamins and antioxidants should be discouraged.

What type, form, dose, and dose-schedule of vitamins and antioxidants should be used in the proposed study?

Type: The type of antioxidant utilized in any given clinical intervention study is extremely important in determining the value of antioxidants in reducing the risk of heart disease.

Most clinical studies designed to study heart disease have utilized only *dietary* antioxidants such as vitamins A, C, E, beta-carotene, and selenium. In some studies other antioxidants derived from fruits and vegetables and herbs have also been used. However, endogenous antioxidants such as glutathione, alpha-lipoic acid, coenzyme Q10, and L-carnitine have *not* been used. Since glutathione is destroyed in the small intestine, n-acetylcysteine (NAC), a glutathione-elevating agent, can and has been used instead.

Both dietary and endogenous antioxidants regulate cellular function in part by different pathways, and they are distributed differently in the cells and organs of the body. Therefore, it's essential to include both dietary and endogenous antioxidants in any multivitamin preparation under consideration for use in a clinical study on heart disease. Most clinical studies pertaining to this area of research have used only one or two dietary antioxidants. Indeed, only one clinical study—to determine the effectiveness of a vitamin preparation containing multiple dietary and endogenous antioxidants, B vitamins, and the appropriate minerals in reducing the risk of heart disease in high-risk populations—has been performed to date.

Form: The form of antioxidant utilized in any given clinical study on heart disease is another very crucial consideration. For example, alpha-tocopheryl succinate was found to be the most effective form of vitamin E in this context (Prasad et al. 2003).

Another finding revealed that the natural form (d) of vitamin E accumulated in various organs of rats more than the synthetic (dl) form of it did (both forms had been administered at the same time) (Ingold et al. 1987). Therefore, natural forms of vitamin E should be added in a multivitamin preparation to be used in heart study.

The natural form of beta-carotene is more effective than the synthetic form of beta-carotene in reducing the incidence of cancer in cell culture (Kennedy and Krinsky 1994). Most major clinical studies on heart disease have utilized the synthetic form of vitamin E or beta-carotene. Vitamin E succinate has never been used in any clinical study on heart disease. This may be due to the fact that many clinicians wrongly believe that all forms of vitamin E produce the same effects.

Dose and dose-schedule: The dose and dose-schedule are also salient factors in determining the effectiveness of antioxidants in reducing the risk of heart disease. Considering that high doses of vitamin A (10,000 IU per day or higher) may produce harmful effects, a lower dose of vitamin A (3,000 IU per day) is recommended. Furthermore, doses of vitamin D that are higher than that currently recommended for adults (400 IU per day) are needed for its optimal beneficial effect. Therefore, the use of a higher dose of vitamin D (800 IU per day or higher) is recommended. Lower doses of antioxidants may reduce only oxidative damage, but higher nontoxic doses of antioxidants may reduce both free radicals and inflammation.

Generally, most clinical studies have utilized antioxidant supplements that have a once-a-day dose-schedule. This dose-schedule may not produce an optimal effect because the biological half-life of vitamins and antioxidants in the plasma vary markedly depending on their extent of solubility in water and fat and their rate of elimination from the body. Thus, taking a multivitamin preparation once a day may create large fluctuations in the levels of vitamins and antioxidants in the body.

For example, a twofold change in the treatment dose of alpha-tocopheryl succinate (vitamin E succinate) caused marked alterations in the expression of gene profiles of neuroblastoma cells in culture. This finding suggests that large fluctuations in the levels of antioxidants in the cells may force them to constantly adjust their genetic activity, which can cause cellular stress over a long period of time. Therefore, a once-a-day dose-schedule may not produce an optimal beneficial effect. Taking a micronutrient preparation twice a day may reduce the degree of this undesirable fluctuation of the levels of vitamins and antioxidants.

What type of the primary and secondary end points (clinical outcomes) should be measured at the end of the study? In all clinical studies with antioxidants, the primary clinical outcomes differed markedly from one study to another. Some studies have utilized symptoms of heart disease. Others have utilized biochemical risk markers associated with the increased chances of developing heart disease. The major primary clinical outcomes in previous studies on antioxidants and heart disease include the following:

1. Myocardial infarction (heart attack)
2. Nonfatal myocardial infarction
3. Death from heart disease
4. Coronary atherosclerosis (stiffening of the arteries to the heart)
5. Cerebral hemorrhage (leakage of blood in the brain)
6. Stenosis in the arteries (narrowing of the arteries)
7. Thrombosis (clot formation in the blood vessels)

The major biological biochemical markers that are considered risk factors of heart disease, determined in previous clinical studies on antioxidants and heart disease, include the following:

1. FMD (endothelial-dependent flow-mediated dilation) of blood vessels (a marker of blood-vessel function)
2. C-reactive protein (CRP)
3. Oxidized LDL cholesterol (damaged by free radicals)
4. Homocysteine
5. Median luminal diameter (MLD) of blood-vessel walls
6. Markers of oxidative stress
7. Markers of chronic inflammation

The secondary clinical outcomes in previous clinical studies on antioxidants and heart disease include the following:

1. Unstable angina (frequent chest pain)
2. Nephropathy (damage to the kidneys)
3. Renal insufficiency (damage to the kidneys)
4. Heart failure

How long should the period of study be so that it can yield meaningful results? In previous clinical studies on antioxidants and heart disease, the period of study varied from three months to ten years. The period of study depends upon the selected clinical outcomes. If the clinical outcomes are markers of oxidative stress and inflammation, a shorter study period is sufficient. However, if the clinical outcomes are major symptoms of heart disease, an observation period of between five and ten years is needed. The differences in clinical outcomes and study period from one study to another are some of the reasons for the inconsistent results that have contributed to the confusion about the value of antioxidants in reducing the risk of heart disease.

THE GENERAL DESIGN OF A TYPICAL CLINICAL INTERVENTION STUDY WITH VITAMINS AND ANTIOXIDANTS

In the typical design of an intervention study, the participants are divided into two groups. One group receives vitamin supplement pills and the other group receives placebo. These placebo pills appear to be similar to the vitamin supplement pill but do not contain any vitamins. The vitamin group is also called the experimental group and the placebo group is called the control group. Patients are randomly selected by a computer to receive vitamins or placebo pills. Studies are considered "blinded" when neither the patients nor the providers of the pills know who is getting which pill. These studies are considered very reliable and are useful in developing public health policy.

Clinical intervention studies pertaining to heart disease are typically categorized as prevention studies and are divided into the categories of primary prevention and secondary prevention. The purpose of primary prevention is to protect healthy individuals from developing heart disease. The purpose of secondary prevention is to stop or slow the progression of risk factors for heart disease. Most clinical studies have tested the effectiveness of antioxidants as secondary prevention;

only a few studies have focused on testing the effectiveness of antioxidants on primary prevention.

Selected clinical studies on the effectiveness of antioxidants on the primary and secondary prevention of heart disease are described next.

PRIMARY PREVENTION STUDIES

The Effect of Vitamin E Alone

In a Harvard study of 39,910 male health professionals, the subset that consumed at least 100 IU of vitamin E per day for a minimum of two years had a 37 percent lower risk of heart disease than those who did not take vitamin E (Rimm et al. 1993).

As referenced earlier another Harvard study of 87,245 healthy nurses, with a follow-up period of eight years, revealed that the relative risk of heart disease was 48 percent lower in those women taking vitamin E supplements that were higher than 100 mg per day for at least two years. An intake of vitamin E obtained only from the diet provided no such protection against heart disease (Stampfer et al. 1993).

The Effect of Multiple Vitamins and Antioxidants

A pilot clinical study was undertaken to test the effectiveness of a commercial preparation of micronutrients containing multiple dietary and endogenous antioxidants* on the risk factors for heart disease in seventy healthy firefighters (who were receiving no heart medication). It was undertaken because of the high number of heart attacks suffered by firefighters on the job. This study was evaluated by Jeff Boone, M.D., of the BraveHeart Program, a division of the Boone Heart Institute in Denver, Colorado.

The study period was for one year. The levels of cholesterols and the coronary artery IMT (width of the wall of the coronary artery) were determined in all participants before the study began and then

---

*The BioArmor Heart Formula from Premier Micronutrient Corporation at www.multimmunity.com.

were measured at six-month and twelve-month intervals. By the end of the study, the results showed that there had been a progressive decrease in LDL cholesterol and an increase in HDL cholesterol. More importantly, the width of the corotid artery wall (IMT; a predictor of coronary health) was reduced when compared to the value observed before vitamin supplementation (Boone and Prasad 2009). To my knowledge no drugs that are currently in use have produced such a biological effect on corotid artery width (unpublished data). If this study were to be confirmed with a larger number of participants, it would have a major impact in reducing the incidence of heart disease by a preparation of multivitamins.

SECONDARY PREVENTION STUDIES

The Effect of Vitamin E Alone

A few clinical studies with vitamin E alone were performed in populations at high risk for developing heart disease, and as expected they all produced inconsistent results varying from no effects, to beneficial effects, to harmful effects.

In the Cambridge Heart Antioxidant Study (CHAOS) (Table 7.1) involving 2,002 patients with proven coronary atherosclerosis, the effectiveness of vitamin E alone on 1,035 patients versus placebo (967 patients) was tested in regard to the risk of dying from heart disease and nonfatal myocardial infarction (MI) as well as nonfatal MI alone. The follow-up period was 510 days. The results showed that vitamin E supplementation markedly reduced the rate of nonfatal MI, however, the number of deaths from heart disease did not significantly change (Stephens et al. 1996).

In a second clinical study involving forty-two patients (thirteen patients with high levels of cholesterol, fourteen tobacco smokers, and fifteen tobacco smokers; Table 7.1.b) who also had high levels of cholesterol, the effectiveness of vitamin E alone on endothelial-dependent flow-mediated dilation (FMD) was evaluated. FMD is a phenomenon wherein an increase in blood flow through a blood vessel causes the vessel to dilate. It is a measure of endothelial cell function that maintains the tone (elasticity) of the blood vessel. Any reduction in FMD may increase the risk of heart disease.

The results of this particular clinical study showed that the levels of autoantibodies created to combat oxidized LDL increased in tobacco smokers with high levels of cholesterol when compared to those found in tobacco smokers alone or patients with high levels of cholesterol alone. Supplementation with vitamin E (alpha-tocopheryl acetate) at a dose of 544 IU improved FMD four months after treatment, but only in smokers with high cholesterol levels (Heitzer et al. 1999). In this study the number of patients was small. A larger number of patients is needed to substantiate this finding.

TABLE 7.1. THE EFFECT OF SUPPLEMENTATION WITH VITAMIN E ALONE IN HIGH-RISK PATIENTS WITH HEART DISEASE

Study	Number of patients	Antioxidant type	Criteria	Follow-up period	Results
a. CHAOS	2,002	Vit. E (d-alpha-T) 400 or 800 IU	Nonfatal MI	510 d	Reduced
b.	15	Vit. E (alpha-TA) 544 IU	FMD	4 months	Improved
c.	100	Vit. E (dl-alpha-T) 1,200 IU	Restenosis	4 months	Reduced

Key:
CHAOS (Cambridge Heart Antioxidant Study)
MI (myocardial infarction)
FMD (endothelial-dependent flow-mediated dilation)
d-alpha-T (natural alpha-tocopherol)
alpha-TA (alpha-tocopheryl acetate)
a. Those with proven atherosclerosis disease
b. Smokers with high levels of cholesterol (hypercholesterolemia)
c. Those who had undergone angioplasty
All vitamins were administered in a once-a-day dose-schedule unless otherwise specified.

In a clinical study (Table 7.1.c) involving one hundred patients who had undergone angioplasty, patients were given either synthetic vitamin E (dl-alpha-tocopherol) at a dose of 1,200 IU per day or placebo in order to evaluate the effectiveness of vitamin E alone in reducing the rate of restenosis (a recurrence of the narrowing of the arteries). The results showed that the incidence of restenosis was 34.6 percent in the vitamin E group; it was 50 percent in the placebo group. This difference of 16 percent was not considered significant (DeMaio et al. 1992). In my opinion a 16 percent reduction is better than no reduction at all; however, a larger number of patients is needed to confirm this result.

Another clinical study referred to as the Alpha-Tocopherol, Beta-Carotene Cancer Prevention (ATBC) study (undertaken from 1985 to 1993) involved 29,133 Finnish male tobacco smokers ages fifty to sixty-nine (Table 7.2). In it the effectiveness of circulating a serum concentration of vitamin E from vitamin supplementation was determined, specifically as it pertained to reducing deaths from heart disease and cancer. Each participant took a pill every day for a period of five to eight years. The pills contained one of the following substances: 50 mg alpha-tocopherol (a form of vitamin E) as dl-alpha-tocopheryl acetate; 20 mg of beta-carotene (a precursor of vitamin A) as all-trans-beta-carotene; both; or a placebo. The results revealed that a higher concentration of serum vitamin E was associated with a reduction in the number of deaths total from cancer, heart disease, and other causes (Table 7.2.a) (Wright et al. 2006).

In the same ATBC study, the effect of oral once-a-day 50 mg supplementation of synthetic dl-alpha-tocopherol, or 20 mg of synthetic beta-carotene, on the risk of heart disease was determined six years after the completion of the trial period of five to eight years. At the beginning of post-trial follow-up, 23,144 men were at risk for a first major heart disease symptom, and 1,255 men with a pre-trial history of heart attack (myocardial infarction) were at risk for a major heart disease symptom.

The results showed that the alpha-tocopherol supplementation did not significantly affect the clinical outcomes in both patient populations, compared to those who received placebo pills (Table 7.2.b). However, the beta-carotene supplementation was shown to increase the risk of major heart disease symptoms, nonfatal myocardial infarction, and fatal coronary heart disease (Table 7.2.e).

This harmful effect of beta-carotene was not observed in the population that had a history of pre-trial heart attack (Tornwall et al. 2004b). It is interesting to note that in the same study population of the ATBC study, vitamin E prevented cerebral infarction (Table 7.2.c) (a condition in which the blood supply to the brain is interrupted), but increased the risk of fatal hemorrhagic strokes (a condition in which a blood vessel in the brain ruptures, causing bleeding) (Table 7.2.f).

In another facet of the ATBC study beta-carotene treatment increased the risk of intracerebral hemorrhage (a condition in which blood vessels in the brain rupture, allowing blood to spread in the brain) (Leppala et al. 2000).

In the same study population, another investigation showed that alpha-tocopherol increased the risk of cerebral infarction (Table 7.2.d). Beta-carotene had no effect (Tornwall et al. 2004a) (Table 7.2.g). The reasons for this discrepancy in the results of these two studies on the same population are unknown.

During a ten-year follow-up of the ATBC trial, 4,647 major cardiac events had occurred in 29,133 subjects who were free of heart disease at the beginning of the trial. The results showed that supplementation with vitamin E alone did not reduce major heart disease symptoms (Knekt et al. 2004).

In another U.S. study of 11,000 people ages sixty-seven or higher, with a follow-up period of six years, it was found that vitamin E supplementation was associated with a 47 percent reduction in deaths from heart disease (Losonczy et al. 1996). A further reduction in the number of deaths was observed in people who were taking vitamin E supplements together with vitamin C.

TABLE 7.2. THE EFFECT OF SUPPLEMENTATION WITH VITAMIN E OR BETA-CAROTENE ALONE IN HIGH-RISK PATIENTS WITH HEART DISEASE

Study	Treatment	End points	Results
a. ATBC	High serum alpha-T	Deaths from all causes	Decreased
b. ATBC	DL-alpha-T 50 mg per day	Heart disease risk	No effect
c. ATBC	DL-alpha-T 50 mg per day	Cerebral infarction risk	Decreased
d. ATBC	DL-alpha-T 50 mg per day	Cerebral infarction risk	Increased
e. ATBC	Synthetic beta-carotene 50 mg per day	Heart disease risk	Increased
f. ATBC	Synthetic beta-carotene 50 mg per day	Fatal hemorrhagic stroke risk	Increased
g. ATBC	Synthetic beta-carotene 50 mg per day	Cerebral infarction risk	No effect
h. HOPE	Natural alpha-T 400 IU per day	All major primary clinical outcomes	No effect
i. HOPE	Natural alpha-T 400 IU per day	Most secondary clinical outcomes	No effect
j. HOPE	Natural alpha-T 400 IU per day	Risk for heart failure/ hospitalization for heart failure	Increased

Key:
ATBC (Alpha-Tocopherol, Beta-Carotene Cancer Prevention) study
HOPE (Heart Outcomes Prevention Evaluation) study
Major clinical outcomes include heart attack, stroke, and death from heart disease. Major secondary clinical outcomes include unstable angina, renal insufficiency, nephropathy, heart failure, and hospitalization for heart failure.
All vitamins were administered in a once-a-day dose-schedule unless otherwise specified.

A clinical study referred to as Heart Outcomes Prevention Evaluation (HOPE) was conducted from December 21, 1993, to April 15, 1999

(Table 7.2.h–j). In it the effectiveness of vitamin E alone on the risk of developing heart disease in high-risk populations was evaluated. This included patients of at least fifty-five years of age with vascular disease or diabetes, many of whom were heavy cigarette smokers. Natural vitamin E at a dose of 400 IU per day was used in this study. The results were analyzed in five separate scientific papers published in peer-reviewed journals. The effectiveness of vitamin E alone was evaluated on four primary clinical outcomes and eight secondary clinical outcomes. The results showed that vitamin E supplementation had no effect on all four primary clinical outcomes, nor did it have any effect on six of the eight secondary clinical outcomes (Yusuf et al. 2000) (Table 7.2.h) (Table 7.2.i). However, another facet of the study showed that vitamin E supplementation increased the risk of two secondary clinical outcomes (heart failure and hospitalization for heart failure) (Table 7.2.j).

In the HOPE trial results that were published in 2000, the primary clinical outcomes were four major heart disease events (heart attack, stroke, death from heart disease, and coronary intima medial thickness), and six secondary clinical outcomes (unstable angina, heart failure, revascularization, amputation, death from heart disease, and complications of diabetes). The results showed that vitamin E supplementation produced no significant effects on the primary or secondary endpoints.

In the analysis published in 2002, the primary clinical outcomes were the same as those that had been published earlier, but the secondary clinical outcomes included an additional outcome: nephropathy (kidney disease). The results showed that vitamin E supplementation alone had no effect on either the primary or secondary clinical outcomes of neuropathy (Lonn et al. 2002).

In the analysis published in 2004, the primary clinical outcomes were the same as those in the study in 2000, but the secondary clinical outcomes included an additional outcome: renal insufficiency, a form of kidney disease. The results showed that vitamin E supplementation alone had no effect on the primary or the secondary clinical outcomes of renal insufficiency (Mann et al. 2004).

In the analysis published in 2005, the primary and secondary clinical outcomes were the same as those published in 2000. The results showed that vitamin E supplementation alone had no effect on the primary and most secondary clinical outcomes. However, it did increase the risk of two secondary clinical outcomes: heart failure and hospitalization for heart failure (Lonn et al. 2005).

The results of the trial as they pertained to heavy tobacco smokers revealed that smoking increased the risk of heart disease and death among this high-risk patient group despite treatment with current medications known to reduce the risk of heart disease (Dagenais et al. 2005).

This is consistent with another independent study in which daily consumption of 800 IU of vitamin E increased the levels of oxidative stress markers in heavy smokers (Weinberg et al. 2001).

These studies suggest that smoking plays a dominant role in increasing the incidence of heart disease and death from heart disease. If these major consequences of heart disease increased despite treatment with current medications to reduce its risk of heart disease in this population of heavy smokers, it's not surprising that the administration of vitamin E alone either had no significant effect on all primary clinical outcomes or most secondary clinical outcomes, or that it increased the risk some of the secondary clinical outcomes (congestive heart failure and hospitalization for heart failure).

It is possible that vitamin E supplementation alone may *increase* the risk of some forms of heart disease in populations that are at a high risk for developing heart disease. This is because, as we have stated earlier, individual antioxidants in high-risk populations, such as tobacco smokers, patients with type 2 diabetes, and patients with a past history of heart attack with defects in the left ventricle, would be oxidized because of the high internal oxidative environment of these patients. In contrast to the effects of vitamin E alone on high-risk populations for developing heart disease, vitamin E supplementation in healthy individuals who had lower levels of oxidative environment did not produce harmful or beneficial effects on the primary or secondary clinical outcomes.

SINGLE AND MULTIPLE AGENT STUDIES

The Effect of Vitamin E Alone or Multiple Antioxidants

Studies on the effectiveness of antioxidants in reducing the biochemical risk factors for heart disease are described in Table 7.3. As you can ascertain from the table, one clinical study involved seventy-two patients (this subset is represented by Table 7.3.a) comprising twenty-three patients with type 2 diabetes with macrovascular complications, (which are defects in larger blood vessels); twenty-four patients with type 2 diabetes without macrovascular complications; and twenty-five matched controls with no diabetes.

In this study the effectiveness of vitamin E alone at a dose of 1,200 IU per day, on blood levels of two inflammation markers—C-reactive protein and interleukin-6—was determined. The results showed that vitamin E supplementation decreased the blood levels of CRP and IL-6 in all three groups (Devaraj and Jialal 2000).

In a clinical study involving thirty-three patients with chronic renal failure (kidney failure) on hemodialysis, chronic renal failure on peritoneal dialysis, and age-sex-matched individuals with no disease, the effectiveness of vitamin E alone at a dose of 800 IU per day on reducing LDL cholesterol oxidation was determined (Table 7.3.b). The results showed that after twelve weeks of vitamin E treatment, the oxidation of LDL cholesterol was reduced in patients with chronic kidney failure, but the beneficial effect was more pronounced in patients with kidney failure on peritoneal dialysis (Islam et al. 2000). In this study the number of patients was small. A larger number of patients is needed to confirm this finding.

In a clinical study involving 182 participants, the effectiveness of a preparation of multivitamins containing B vitamins and antioxidants on reducing the levels of homocysteine and the oxidation of LDL cholesterol was determined (Table 7.3.c). The results showed that multivitamin supplementations reduced the levels of homocysteine and LDL cholesterol oxidation (Earnest et al. 2003).

TABLE 7.3. THE EFFECT OF VITAMIN E ALONE OR MULTIPLE ANTIOXIDANTS ON BIOCHEMICAL RISK FACTORS IN HIGH-RISK PATIENTS WITH HEART DISEASE

No. of patients	Antioxidant	Criteria of study	Follow-up period	Results
a. 72	Vit. E	1,200 IU CRP, IL-6	5 months	Reduced
b. 33	Vit. E (d-αT) 800 IU	LDL oxidation	12 weeks	Reduced
c. 182	Multivitamins	Homocysteine, LDL oxidation	6 months	Reduced

Key:

a. Patients with type 2 diabetes

b. Patients with chronic renal failure (kidney failure) undergoing peritoneal dialysis or hemodialysis

c. Patients with hypercholesterolemia (high levels of cholesterol), CRP (C-reactive protein), IL-6 (interleukin-6)

The Effect of Vitamin C Alone

In a clinical study involving 175 patients who were going to have heart surgery, supplementation with vitamin C before and after surgery reduced the incidence of atrial fibrillation (rapid, irregular heartbeat) following the surgery, decreased the time needed for the return to a normal heartbeat, and decreased the length of the hospital stay (Papoulidis et al. 2011). A protein called CD40L is located on many cells; however, 95 percent of circulating CD40L is located on platelets. Levels of CD40L are elevated in patients undergoing coronary stent procedures. This protein initiates the inflammatory response and thus plays a role in the development of atherosclerosis.

In a clinical study involving fifty-six patients undergoing elective coronary stent procedures, the effectiveness of vitamin C infusion on the plasma levels of CD40L was tested. The results showed that infusion of vitamin C reduced the plasma levels of CD40L (Pignatelli et al. 2011).

The Effect of a Combination of Vitamin E and Vitamin C

The Women's Angiographic Vitamin and Estrogen (WAVE) trial was conducted on postmenopausal women suffering from progressive heart disease. These women had at least one coronary artery that revealed coronary stenosis (narrowing) at 15 to 75 percent of coronary in a baseline coronary angiography. The trial was conducted from July 1997 to January 2002. Antioxidants (400 IU of vitamin E and 500 mg of vitamin C twice daily) were administered orally (Table 7.4.d) (Table 7.4.e) (Table 7.4.f).

The primary clinical outcome was a change in the minimum luminal diameter (MLD) of blood vessels. The results showed that in postmenopausal women who had progressive heart disease, supplementation with two dietary antioxidants (vitamin E and vitamin C) produced no benefits (Table 7.4.e).

In results of the same WAVE trial published later, in 2005, treatment with a combination of vitamin E and vitamin C did not improve flow-mediated dilation (FMD) (Table 7.4.e) (Kelemen et al. 2005). The results from the subgroup of patients with haptoglobin (hp) alleles (a type of gene) showed that a combined treatment with vitamin E and vitamin C increased MLD compared to the group receiving placebo pills (Table 7.4.f).

This effect was more pronounced in women with diabetes compared to those who did not have diabetes (Levy et al. 2004).

Increased oxidative stress is found in patients with heart transplants, which may enhance the development of coronary atherosclerosis. This idea was tested in a clinical study involving forty patients (nineteen patients on vitamin supplement and twenty patients on placebo pills). The effects of a combination of vitamin E (400 IU twice a day) and vitamin C (500 mg twice a day) on the development of atherosclerosis were determined, in these patients, from zero to two years after they had undergone heart transplants (Table 7.4.a). After one year of treatment with vitamins, the progression of atherosclerosis had been reduced in these patients (Fang et al. 2002). In this study the number of patients was small. A larger number of patients is needed to confirm this finding.

In a clinical study involving 520 men and women ages forty-five to sixty-nine who had high levels of cholesterol (hypercholesterolemia), the effect of a combination of vitamin E and slow-release vitamin C on the progression of carotid atherosclerosis, a risk factor for heart disease, was determined (Table 7.4.b). The results showed that after six years of follow-up, vitamin supplement reduced carotid atherosclerosis by about 26 percent (33 percent in men and 14 percent in women) (Salonen 2002).

TABLE 7.4. THE EFFECT OF VITAMIN E IN COMBINATION WITH VITAMIN C IN HIGH-RISK PATIENTS WITH HEART DISEASE

No. of patients	Antioxidant	Criteria of study	Follow-up period	Results
a. 40	Vit. E 400 IU + Vit. C 500 mg	Coronary atherosclerosis	1 year	Reduced
b. 520	Vit. E + slow-release Vit. C.	Atherosclerosis	6 years	Reduced
c. 20	Vit. E 88 IU + Vit. C 1 g	FMD	6 hours	Increased
d. WAVE	Vit. E 400 IU + Vit. C 500 mg	MLD	No effect	
e. WAVE	Vit. E 400 IU + Vit. C 500 mg	FMD	No effect	
f. WAVE	Vit. E 400 IU + Vit. C 500 mg	MLD	Increased*	

Key:
WAVE (Women's Angiographic Vitamin and Estrogen) study
FMD (endothelial-dependent flow-mediated dilation)
LDL-C (LDL-cholesterol)
MLD (median luminal diameter)
FMD (flow-mediated dilation)
*Patients with haptoglobin allele showing beneficial effect
a. cardiac transplant individuals
b. individuals with hypercholesterolemia
c. normal individuals consuming high-fat meals

Increased oxidative stress, endothelial function defects (reduced FMD), and stiffness of the arteries are found in patients with hypertension (high blood pressure). A clinical study involving thirty men with hypertension was performed in order to evaluate the effectiveness of a combined treatment with vitamin E (400 IU) and vitamin C (1,000 mg) on increased oxidative stress, reduced FMD, and stiffness of the arteries. After eight weeks the group that had been treated with vitamins showed improvement in arterial stiffness and FMD compared to the group receiving placebo pills (Plantinga et al. 2007). These beneficial effects were associated with increased plasma levels of antioxidants and decreased oxidative stress. In this study the number of patients was small. A larger number of patients is needed to confirm this finding.

Increased oxidative stress and oxidized LDL cholesterol impair the functioning of endothelial cells by reducing nitric oxide (NO), which is necessary for the dilation of blood vessels. In a clinical study involving thirty subjects, the effectiveness of a combination of vitamin E (800 IU) and vitamin C (1,000 mg) on endothelial cell function was tested. After six months of treatment, the group that had been treated with vitamins showed no improvement in coronary artery or brachial artery endothelial function (FMD) (Kinlay et al. 2004).

Similar results were obtained in another clinical study with eighteen non-smoking and non-diabetic subjects who were treated with a combination of 400 IU of vitamin E, 500 mg of vitamin C, 12 mg of beta-carotene or 800 IU of vitamin E, 1,000 mg of vitamin C, and 24 mg of beta-carotene for a period of three months (McKechnie et al. 2002). The patient populations in these two studies did not belong to high-risk populations for developing heart disease and thus are different from those studies in which beneficial effects on endothelial function were noted after treatment with vitamin E and vitamin C. In addition the number of patients in these two studies was small. Given these concerns a larger number of patients is needed to confirm this specific finding.

Increased oxidative stress is involved in causing defects in endothelial function (defects in blood-vessel dilation) and acute myocardial infarction (acute heart attack) with or without diabetes. It was thought that supplementation with antioxidants might be beneficial to these patients. A clinical study referred to as the Myocardial Infarction and Vitamins (MIVIT) study recruited 800 patients with acute myocardial infarction with or without diabetes to test the effectiveness of a combination of vitamin E and vitamin C in reducing death from heart disease. About 15 percent of those who had acute myocardial infarction had diabetes. The results showed that vitamin E treatment reduced death from heart disease from 14 percent to 5 percent in patients with acute myocardial infarction who also had diabetes, but this beneficial effect was not seen in patients with acute myocardial infarction who did *not* have diabetes (Jaxa-Chamiec et al. 2009).

These studies on the effectiveness of two dietary antioxidants (vitamin E and vitamin C) produced inconsistent results in populations that are at a high risk for developing heart disease. Therefore, we do not recommend the use of one or two dietary antioxidants in the prevention of heart disease.

CLINICAL OUTCOME STUDIES

The Effect of N-acetylcysteine and Alpha-Lipoic Acid

Like dietary antioxidants, endogenous antioxidants such as the glutathione-elevating agent n-acetylcysteine (NAC) and alpha-lipoic acid produced inconsistent results when used individually. In a study with one hundred patients, prophylactic use of NAC in patients undergoing coronary artery bypass grafting did not improve clinical outcomes or biochemical markers (El-Hamamsy et al. 2007).

However, in another study involving forty patients, prophylactic administration of NAC attenuated myocardial oxidative stress in the heart of patients undergoing cardiopulmonary bypass (Tossios et al. 2003).

In a short-term (eight-week) study involving thirty-six patients, an oral administration of NAC and alpha-lipoic acid increased brachial artery diameter and reduced arterial stiffness. It also decreased systolic blood pressure in patients with heart disease (McMackin et al. 2007).

Atrial fibrillation (rapid, irregular heartbeat) is common after heart surgery. Increased evidence suggests that elevated oxidative stress plays a significant role in the development of atrial fibrillation. A review of eight clinical trials involving 578 patients who were going to have heart surgery suggested that pre-treatment with NAC reduced the incidence of atrial fibrillation after heart surgery compared to those who did not receive NAC. It had no effect on the length of the hospital stay (Gu et al. 2012).

The Effect of Coenzyme Q10 Alone

Plasma levels of coenzyme Q10 decrease in patients with advanced chronic heart failure. It is not known whether coenzyme Q10 supplementation can reduce the symptoms of chronic heart failure. In a clinical study with twenty-three patients (twenty men and three women) with stable chronic heart failure, the effectiveness of coenzyme Q10 at an oral dose of 100 mg per day with or without supervised training (five times per week) on endothelial function and left ventricle contractility (blood-pumping capacity of the ventricle) was tested. The results showed that after four weeks of treatment with coenzyme Q10 supplementation, there was improved endothelial function (coronary FMD) and left ventricles contractility in patients with chronic heart failure, without any toxic side effects. The combination of coenzyme Q10 and exercise was more effective than the individual agents (Belardinelli et al. 2006).

Defects in endothelial and mitochondrial function were found in patients with heart disease. In a clinical study involving fifty-six patients with heart disease (ischemic left ventricular systolic dysfunction, e.g., a pumping defect of the left ventricle), the effectiveness of coenzyme Q10 at an oral dose of 300 mg per day on mitochondrial and ventricular dysfunction (a defect in FMD) was tested. The results showed that after eight weeks of treatment, coenzyme Q10 improved mitochondrial function and brachial artery FMD (Dai et al. 2011).

The Effect of Resveratrol Alone

Several epidemiological and experimental studies have shown that drinking a moderate amount of wine, particularly red wine, reduced the risks of heart disease, stroke, and peripheral vascular disease (Bertelli and Das 2009; Penumathsa and Maulik 2009). The protective effects of wine were primarily due to the presence of antioxidants (primarily resveratrol) found in grape skin and the proanthocyanidins that are found in grape seed. Most studies on the effectiveness of resveratrol in reducing the risk of heart disease have been performed in animals.

White wine also reduced the incidence of heart disease in animal models. This effect of white wine was primarily due to the presence of the antioxidants tyrosol and hydroxytyrosol (Dudley et al. 2008).

These antioxidants increased the functions of mitochondria. Resveratrol reduced infarct size and prevented mitochondrial swelling in the heart muscle cells of rats during reperfusion injury (injury caused by a rapid blood flow to the areas previously rendered ischemic by coronary artery blockage) (Xi et al. 2009).

Resveratrol also protected heart muscle cells against hydrogen peroxide (H_2O_2)-induced apoptosis (cell death) (Yu et al. 2009). Administration of resveratrol significantly reduced myocardial infarction-induced ventricular tachycardia and ventricular fibrillation.

In addition infract size and mortality were reduced in resveratrol-treated rats (Chen et al. 2008).

COMBINATION STUDIES

Results of Previous Clinical Studies on Antioxidants in Combination with Cholesterol-Lowering Drugs

A summary of clinical studies in high-risk patients treated with antioxidants in combination with cholesterol-lowering drugs is described in Table 7.5. The number, type, dose, and dose-schedules of antioxidants, patient populations, observation periods, and clinical outcomes of the studies were different. In seven patients with an excess of cholesterol (hypercholesterolemia), vitamin E supplementation (300 IU per day), together with simvastatin for an eight-week period, improved endothelial-dependent flow-mediated dilation (FMD). It also improved endothelial-dependent nitroglycerine-mediated dilation (NMD) in the brachial arteries of patients with hypercholesterolemia more than that produced by simvastatin alone (Neunteufl et al. 1998) (Table 7.5).

TABLE 7.5. THE EFFECT OF ANTIOXIDANTS IN COMBINATION WITH CHOLESTEROL-LOWERING DRUGS IN HIGH-RISK PATIENTS WITH HEART DISEASE

Study	No. of patients	Clinical outcome antioxidant +	Cholesterol-lowering drug	Follow-up	Results
a. ——	7	Vit. E 300 IU + Simvastatin	FMD, NMD	8 weeks	Improved
b. HPS	20,500	Vit E. 650 mg; Vit. C 250 mg; Beta-carotene 20 mg	Cardiac events	5.5 years	No better than drug alone

Key:
HPS (Heart Protection Study): Elderly patients with diabetes, individuals with low baseline cholesterol, and those who previously had occlusive non-coronary vascular disease
FMD (endothelial-dependent flow-mediated dilation)
NMD (endothelial-independent nitroglycerine-mediated dilation)
a. individuals with hypercholesterolemia
All vitamins were administered in a once-a-day dose-schedule unless otherwise specified.

The Heart Protection Study (HPS) (Collins et al. 2002) included 20,500 patients with a high risk of developing heart disease. The high-risk individuals included elderly patients with diabetes, individuals on statins, and those who had a previous history of occlusive non-coronary vascular disease. The effectiveness of supplementation with antioxidants (vitamin E 650 mg, vitamin C 250 mg, and beta-carotene 20 mg), together with simvastatin, on deaths from all causes (total mortality), deaths from vascular disease (vascular mortality), major heart disease events, and stroke was tested for a period of five and a half years. The results showed that treatment with antioxidants (a combination of vitamin C, vitamin E, and beta-carotene) did not interfere with the effectiveness of statins in reducing the risk of events that were related to heart disease. Antioxidant treatment did not reduce the risk of heart disease (Table 7.5.b).

In the HDL Atherosclerosis Treatment Study (HATS), the effects of dietary antioxidants in combination with cholesterol-lowering drugs on stenosis and HDL cholesterol were evaluated in high-risk heart disease patients with low HDL cholesterol (Brown et al. 2001; Cheung et al. 2001). Dietary antioxidants included 1,000 mg of vitamin C, 800 IU of vitamin E as d-α-tocopherol, 25 mg of natural beta-carotene, and 100 μg of selenium per day, given together with simvastatin-niacin in a subset of patients with low levels of HDL cholesterol (Table 7.6). The results revealed that the niacin-induced elevation of HDL cholesterol was reduced by antioxidant supplements (Table 7.6.a) (Table 7.6.b).

The same group of investigators using the same formulation reported that antioxidants reduced the degree of proximal artery stenosis in comparison with the placebo group, which did not receive any drug or antioxidants. However, a combination of simvastatin-niacin and antioxidant supplementation was less effective than the simvastatin-niacin treatment alone in reducing the degree of stenosis. Yet this conclusion appears premature. This is due to the fact that the sample size for this portion of the study was only forty patients per group, which is considered too small to make a definitive conclusion.

In addition percent variation around the average value, especially of simvastatin-niacin and simvastatin-niacin plus the antioxidant groups, was very high (557 to 800 percent). These levels of variation around the average value would not allow any definitive conclusions regarding the effectiveness of antioxidants in improving simvastatin-niacin therapy. Furthermore, endogenous antioxidants such as glutathione-elevating agents (n-acetylcysteine), alpha-lipoic acid, coenzyme Q10, and L-carnitine were not included in the preparation of dietary antioxidants. It is interesting to note that in the same population of HATS, antioxidants in combination with simvastatin-niacin did not alter the plasma levels of markers of cholesterol synthesis and absorption compared to simvastatin-niacin alone (Table 7.6.c) (Matthan et al. 2003). Thus, at this time, it is not possible to conclude that antioxidant supplementation in combination with simvastatin-niacin therapy enhances the degree of stenosis more than that produced by drug therapy alone.

TABLE 7.6. THE EFFECT OF MULTIPLE DIETARY ANTIOXIDANTS IN COMBINATION WITH CHOLESTEROL-LOWERING DRUGS IN HIGH-RISK PATIENTS WITH HEART DISEASE

Study	No. of patients	Antioxidant + cholesterol-lowering drug	Criteria of study	Follow-up	Results
a. HATS	160	Vit. E 800 IU, Vit.C 1 g, beta-carotene 25 mg, selenium 100 mcg + Simvastatin + niacin	Stenosis	3 year	Reduced drug effectiveness, but was more effective than control without antioxidant
b. HATS	153	Same antioxidants + Simvastatin + niacin	HDL	1 year	Reduced drug effectiveness
c. HATS	153	Same antioxidants + Simvastatin + niacin	Markers of cholesterol synthesis and absorption	No effect	

Key:
HATS (HDL Atherosclerosis Treatment Study)
HDL (high-density lipoprotein cholesterol)
a. Patients with heart disease who had low HDL and normal LDL levels
All vitamins were administered in a once-a-day dose-schedule unless otherwise specified.

TABLE 7.7. THE EFFECT OF MULTIPLE DIETARY
ANTIOXIDANTS ALONE OR IN COMBINATION WITH
SIMVASTATIN-NIACIN ON THE PROGRESSION OF STENOSIS
(THE NARROWING OF A CORONARY ARTERY)
IN HIGH-RISK PATIENTS WITH HEART DISEASE

Treatments	Percent progression of stenosis	Percent variation around average value
Placebo group	3.9 ± 5.2	133
Antioxidant group	1.8 ± 4.2	233
Simvastatin-niacin group	0.4 ± 2.8	700
Simvastatin-niacin + antioxidant group	0.7 ± 3.2	457

Antioxidant group: Dietary antioxidants included 800 IU of
vitamin E, 1,000 mg of vitamin C, 25 mg of beta-carotene,
and 100 mcg of selenium

One hundred sixty patients were recruited for this study. The number of patients per group was probably only forty. This number is too small for any meaningful conclusions to be drawn. In addition percent variation around the average value, especially of simvastatin-niacin and simvastatin-niacin plus antioxidant groups, was very high.

STUDIES WITH B VITAMINS, OMEGA-3 FATTY ACIDS, AND ADDITIONAL STUDIES ON THE RISK OF HEART DISEASE

The Effect of B Vitamins Alone

Supplements of certain B vitamins (B_6, B_{12}, and folic acid) reduce homocysteine levels; therefore, it was thought that reducing the level of homocysteine may reduce the risk of developing heart disease. In view of the fact that the effect of homocysteine is mediated by free radicals (Perez-de-Arce et al. 2005), a reduction in homocysteine alone may not be sufficient to reduce the risk of heart disease. In fact, clinical studies with B vitamins showed that supplementation with B vitamins alone either increased the risk factors for heart disease or had no effect.

In a clinical study involving 3,749 men and women who had an acute myocardial infarction (heart attack) seven days before the start of the experiment, the effectiveness of B vitamins in reducing the risk of recurrent myocardial infarction, stroke, and sudden death from heart disease was tested. The patients were divided as follows: (a) a group receiving 0.8 mg folic acid and 0.4 mg B_{12}; (b) a group receiving 40 mg of B_6 alone; (c) a group receiving 0.8 mg folic, 0.4 mg B_{12}, and 40 mg of B_6; and (d) a group receiving placebo (placebo pills) (Table 7.8). The results showed that homocysteine levels in the plasma decreased in the group that had been treated with B vitamins, but there was no significant difference in recurrent myocardial infarction, stroke, or sudden death from heart disease between groups (a) and (b) when compared to those who had received placebo pills (group d). However, group (c) showed an increased risk of developing of all three primary clinical outcomes (Bonaa et al. 2006).

In a clinical study involving 5,522 patients ages fifty-five or older who had vascular disease or diabetes, the effectiveness of B vitamins on recurrent myocardial infarction, stroke, or sudden death from heart disease was tested. Patients were administered a daily oral combination of 2.5 mg of folic acid, 50 mg of vitamin B_6, and 1 mg of vitamin B_{12} for an average period of five years. The results showed that plasma levels of homocysteine decreased in the group that had been treated with vitamins, but had no significant effect on three primary clinical outcomes (myocardial infarction, stroke, and death from heart disease) (Lonn et al. 2006).

Using the same patient population, it was demonstrated that the incidence of venous thrombosis (clots in the veins) or pulmonary embolism (a sudden blockage of a pulmonary artery) in the group that had been treated with vitamins was similar to that found in the placebo group (Table 7.8) (Ray 2007).

TABLE 7.8. THE EFFECT OF B VITAMINS ALONE ON MAJOR CLINICAL OUTCOMES IN HIGH-RISK PATIENTS WITH HEART DISEASE

Patient type	Vitamin treatment	End points	Results
a. 3,749 patients with one MI	Folic acid 0.8 mg, Vit. B_6 40 mg, Vit. B_{12} 0.4 mg	Recurrent MI, stroke, death	Increase
b. 5,522 patients with vascular disease or diabetes	Folic acid 2.5 mg, Vit. B_6 50 mg, Vit. B_{12} 1 mg	MI, stroke, death	No effect
c. Same 5,522 patients with vascular disease or diabetes	Folic acid 2.5 mg, Vit. B_6 50 mg, Vit. B_{12} 1 mg	Venous thrombosis	No effect
d. 3,680 patients with non-disabling cerebral infarction	Multiple vitamins* and high-dose or low-dose B vitamins†	MI, stroke, death	No effect

Key:
MI = myocardial infarction (heart attack)
*An FDA reference daily intake of other vitamins.
†High-dose B vitamins (2.5 mg of folic acid, 25 mg of vitamin B_6, and 0.4 mg of vitamin B_{12}); low-dose B vitamins (20 mcg of folic acid, 200 mcg of vitamin B_6, and 6 mcg of vitamin B_{12})

In a clinical study involving 3,680 patients with non-disabling cerebral infarction, the effectiveness of B vitamins on recurrent cerebral infarction (primary clinical outcome) and heart disease events, and death from heart disease, was tested (Toole et al. 2004). The experimental design for this study was totally different from those described in the three aforementioned studies. All patients received medical and surgical care plus a daily supplementation with a multivitamin containing the U.S. Food and Drug Administration's reformed daily intake of other vitamins. They were also randomly assigned to daily doses of high or low doses of B vitamins.

The patients were divided into two groups. One group received high doses of B vitamins (25 mg of vitamin B_6, 0.4 mg of vitamin B_{12}, and 2.5 mg of folic acid), and the other group received low doses of B vitamins (200 mcg of vitamin B6, 6 mcg of vitamin B12, and 20 mcg of folic acid). They were followed for a period of two years (Table 7.8). The results showed that plasma levels of homocysteine decreased more in the high-dose group than in the low-dose group, but B vitamin treatment had no effect on primary or secondary clinical outcomes.

Based on the results of these studies, two conclusions can be made: (1) high-dose B vitamins should not be recommended to patients who have had one myocardial infarction, and (2) for other high-risk heart disease populations, supplementation with folic acid, vitamin B6, and vitamin B12 had no effect on the incidence of heart attack, stroke, or death from heart disease.

If increased levels of homocysteine are a risk factor for the development of heart disease, why didn't vitamin B supplements, which decreased the levels of homocysteine by about 25 percent, reduce the risk of heart disease? This could have been because the designs of the clinical studies discussed herein did not take into account the fact that homocysteine causes damage to endothelial cells by free radicals. Therefore, a modest reduction in homocysteine levels is not expected to have any significant effect on any of the primary clinical outcomes such as myocardial infarction, stroke, and death from heart disease. In addition other risk factors—such as increased oxidative stress generated by mechanisms other than homocysteine levels, chronic inflammation, and the oxidation of LDL cholesterol—were not affected by supplementation with B vitamins alone. Hence, the addition of antioxidants may be necessary to demonstrate the beneficial effect of B vitamins on reducing the incidence of heart disease.

The Effect of Omega-3 Fatty Acids Alone

Omega-3 fatty acids are essential fatty acids consisting of three major types including alpha-linolenic acid (ALA), eicosapentaenoic acid (EPA), and docosahexaenoic acid (DHA). ALA is primarily obtained from the diet, whereas EPA and DHA are obtained from fatty fish and also are formed from ALA in the body. Several reviews on the efficacy of omega-3 fatty acids have revealed that supplementation with omega-3 from fish or omega-3 capsules reduced the risk of cardiac events in patients with heart disease (He 2009; Holub 2009; Lavie et al. 2009; Lee et al. 2009; Marchioli et al. 2009).

Chronic kidney disease is associated with an increased risk of heart disease. In a clinical study involving eighty-five non-diabetic patients with chronic kidney disease, it was observed that supplementation with omega-3 fatty acids reduced blood pressure, heart rate, and triglycerides (Mori et al. 2009).

A review of the literature has confirmed that supplementation with omega-3 fatty acids significantly improved arterial hypertension (Cicero et al. 2009).

Omega-3 fatty acids exhibit a wide range of biological activities (Dimitrow and Jawien 2009; Simopoulos 2008). They serve to:

1. Regulate FMD (a flow-mediated dilation of the blood vessels) and renal sodium excretion
2. Reduce angiotensin-converting enzyme activity
3. Enhance production of endothelial nitric oxide
4. Activate the parasympathetic nervous system
5. Reduce inflammation and platelet aggregation
6. Improve endothelial cell function

These studies are convincing in suggesting that supplementation with omega-3 fatty acids appears to be useful in most cases of heart disease.

The Effect of Garlic, Flavonols, and Curcumin

A review of several studies has shown that an increased intake of garlic may reduce blood pressure in patients with elevated blood pressure, but not in those individuals whose blood pressure is normal (Reinhart et al. 2008).

A review of several studies suggests that flavonols such as quercetin reduce blood pressure, atherosclerosis, and endothelial damage. They also protect the heart against damage produced by a reduced oxygen supply (Perez-Vizcaino and Duarte 2010).

Curcumin, a polyphenol that is derived from the spice turmeric, reduced some risks of heart disease in animal studies and in limited human studies.

CONCLUDING REMARKS

Laboratory studies on heart disease measuring the effect of a single antioxidant have shown a beneficial effect in reducing its risk. However, human studies of high-risk patients, designed to measure the effect of individual dietary antioxidants—including vitamin E, beta-carotene, B vitamins, resveratrol, or omega-3 fatty acids alone—have produced beneficial effects, no effects, or harmful effects. The harmful effects produced may be due to the fact that oxidation of the individual anti-oxidant takes place in the high internal oxidative environments of those at high risk for heart disease and, instead of acting in a therapeutic fashion as an antioxidant, becomes a harmful prooxidant instead. If the same antioxidant is present in a multivitamin preparation, the presence of other antioxidants would prevent the oxidation of individual antioxidants. Therefore, we do not recommend consumption of a single antioxidant, B vitamins, or omega-3 fatty acids alone for normal populations or populations that are at a high risk for developing heart disease.

Supporting this finding that argues in support of the administration of a multivitamin supplement for high-risk populations is another finding. This second finding has determined that the administration of a commercial supplement containing several dietary and endogenous antioxidants, B vitamins, and appropriate minerals, to a population of high-risk firefighters, was helpful in reducing their risk of developing heart disease.

Be this as it may, the fact that human studies of high-risk patients utilizing a single antioxidant have produced variable results as noted above points to the need for studies that are better designed. Earlier in the chapter we discussed all of the criteria that should be considered when undertaking the design of a clinical intervention study. In the next chapter we will examine this issue more closely. As we shall see current failings in the study of heart disease have much to do with this lack of regard for the tenets of a well-designed clinical study.

8 Clinical Studies to Date

A Flawed Methodology

Although there is a uniformity of opinion among the scientific and medical communities about the value of changing one's diet and lifestyle in order to reduce the incidence of heart disease, there is no such agreement about the value of vitamins and antioxidant supplements in regard to this issue.

Several well-designed clinical studies have been performed to test the effectiveness of a single antioxidant, B vitamin, or omega-3 fatty acids in reducing the risk of heart disease. The results of these studies varied from some transient benefits, to no effects, to harmful effects, depending upon the type of antioxidants employed and the clinical outcomes.

This issue has been discussed in detail in the previous chapter, but bears summarization here. In a clinical trial referred to as the HOPE trial, vitamin E supplementation had no effect on four major primary clinical outcomes (heart attack, stroke, death from heart disease, and coronary intima medial thickness). Nor did it have any effect on six out of eight secondary clinical outcomes (unstable angina, heart failure, revascularization, amputation, diabetic complications, nephropathy, a form of kidney disease, and renal insufficiency). However, vitamin E appeared to increase the risk of two secondary clinical outcomes (heart failure and hospitalization for heart failure) in one study. The major conclusion of this scientific report *should* have been that vitamin E alone should not be administered to those who are at high risk for developing heart disease, because this treatment may be ineffective or even harmful in some high-risk populations.

It is incorrect to think that the effects of a single antioxidant on heart disease prevention would produce the same effects as those produced by multivitamins and antioxidants instead. Unfortunately, this scientific report derived from the HOPE trial has become a major reason why physicians do not recommend multivitamin supplements for reducing the risk of heart disease. No study on heart disease has been performed to evaluate the effectiveness of a vitamin preparation containing *multiple* dietary antioxidants (the B vitamins, vitamin C, vitamin E, beta-carotene, selenium) and endogenous antioxidants (alpha-lipoic acid, n-acetylcysteine, a glutathione-elevating agent, coenzyme Q10, and L-carnitine), vitamin D, and appropriate minerals including selenium. Nevertheless, many in the scientific and medical communities believe that a multivitamin preparation may produce results similar to those produced by a single agent. Therefore, they don't feel comfortable recommending a multiple combination of vitamins and antioxidants to their patients with heart disease.

The question arises: What is the basis for their beliefs and how can the issue be resolved? This chapter describes why clinical studies with antioxidants have failed to yield consistent beneficial results in reducing the risk of heart disease, why controversies continue to exist among most physicians and health care professionals, and what should be done to resolve these conflicts.

WHY CURRENT RECOMMENDATIONS ARE NOT HAVING THE DESIRED OUTCOMES

Lack of Adherence to All of the Criteria

In order for progress to be made in preventing and treating heart disease, there should be an accord among treating physicians as to treatment protocols. A first step in obtaining such an accord might be to ensure that the methodology used to derive study results is thoroughly adhered to and standardized as much as possible. To examine this point in a comprehensive fashion, we will revisit the criteria for a successful intervention study as outlined in the previous chapter in order to more specifically pinpoint where current failings may lie.

1. What are the appropriate patient populations for the study of heart disease?
2. What are the blood levels of the markers of oxidative stress and chronic inflammation in patients selected for the study?
3. How many vitamins and antioxidants (single vs. multiple) should be used in the proposed study?
4. What form, type, dose, and dose-schedule of vitamins and antioxidants should be used in the proposed study?
5. What type of the primary and secondary end points (clinical outcomes) should be measured at the end of the study?
6. How long should the study period be in order that it yields meaningful results?

In the study designs of all previous clinical studies published to date, questions 1, 5, and 6 were taken into account, but questions 2, 3, and 4 were either not carefully considered or were often ignored. This may have contributed to conflicting results on the effectiveness of antioxidant supplementation in reducing the risk of heart disease. Inconsistent results obtained from the use of a single antioxidant, B vitamins, or omega-3 fatty acids alone in patients at high risk for developing heart disease are primarily responsible for the continued doubts about the value of vitamins and antioxidants in this regard. Let's now more closely examine some of these concerns, as well as explore a few additional ones.

High Internal Oxidative Environment in High-Risk Populations

Most clinical studies have utilized a single antioxidant, primarily vitamin E, to evaluate the effectiveness of antioxidants in reducing the risk of heart disease in high-risk populations. However, as we know, high-risk populations such as heavy tobacco smokers and patients with diabetes have a high internal oxidative environment due to the production of excessive amounts of free radicals in the body and the depletion of antioxidants from the body.

Single antioxidants such as vitamin E or beta-carotene are gradually oxidized in the presence of a high oxidative environment and then act as a harmful prooxidant rather than as an antioxidant. If the same single antioxidant is present in a vitamin preparation containing *multiple* dietary and endogenous antioxidants, however, the conversion of an antioxidant to a prooxidant form would not occur because other antioxidants would prevent this from happening.

Reliance on the Results of Animal Studies for the Design of Human Studies

Another contributing factor as to why current recommendations are not having the desired effect is the fact that the clinical studies that have been done to date have relied heavily on the results of animal studies, which have consistently shown that the administration of a single antioxidant reduced the risk for heart disease from chemical-induced sources or from fat-based sources in the diet. However, from the results of these studies alone, one should not conclude that similar results (utilizing a single antioxidant) would be obtained in humans. It should always be remembered that animal studies with antioxidants provide *only a guide* with respect to their effectiveness in reducing the risk of heart disease in humans. The effective dose, dose-schedule, safety, and period of observation that are used in animal studies with antioxidants cannot be used in the design of human studies.

This is due to the fact that the extent of effectiveness, absorption, metabolism (turnover), excretion (elimination), and toxicity of antioxidants in animals are totally different from those in humans. In addition and as we have mentioned previously, most mammals make their own vitamin C. Humans, however, rely on the diet for vitamin C. The presence of endogenous vitamin C in most animals can influence the effectiveness of a multivitamin preparation in reducing the risk of heart disease.

THE RATIONALE FOR USING A VITAMIN PREPARATION CONTAINING MULTIPLE DIETARY AND ENDOGENOUS ANTIOXIDANTS IN CLINICAL STUDIES

There are several reasons for using a multivitamin preparation in clinical studies that examine the risk of heart disease and how best to reduce the incidence of it. As we know increased oxidative stress, chronic inflammation, and homocysteine levels are key factors that participate in the development and progression of heart disease. Therefore, the use of antioxidants that decrease oxidative stress and chronic inflammation, and B vitamins that decrease homocysteine levels, must be used together in order to reduce these risk factors at the same time. Multiple antioxidants act in a synergistic (more than an additive effect) manner to influence the disease process.*

It is known that different types of free radicals are produced in the body. The body also has multiple dietary and endogenous antioxidants to destroy these free radicals when they are produced in excessive amounts. Each antioxidant has a different affinity for each of these free radicals, depending upon the cellular environment. The level of oxygen pressure varies within cells and tissues. Vitamin E, for instance, is more effective in neutralizing free radicals in an internal environment that is marked by reduced oxygen pressure. Beta-carotene and vitamin A are

---

*The reference for this section has been provided in a review (Prasad, 2011).

more effective in an internal environment marked by higher oxygen pressure.

Vitamin C is necessary to protect cellular components immersed in water against free radical damage. Carotenoids and vitamins A and E protect cellular components in lipid (fat-soluble) environments. Vitamin C also plays a necessary role in maintaining cellular levels of vitamin E by recycling damaged vitamin E (oxidized) to the antioxidant (reduced) form. The form and type of vitamin E used are also important considerations when seeking to improve its beneficial effects. It is known that various organs of rats selectively absorb the natural form of vitamin E; therefore, the natural form of vitamin E, alpha tocopheryl-succinate (vitamin E succinate), is recommended for inclusion in multivitamin preparations utilized in clinical studies.

The natural forms of vitamin E and beta-carotene are more effective than their synthetic counterparts. For example, natural beta-carotene reduced radiation-induced cancer formation in mammalian cells in culture, but the synthetic form of beta-carotene did not. Antioxidants are distributed differently in various organs and even within the same cells. Selenium, a cofactor of glutathione peroxidase, acts as an antioxidant. Therefore, selenium supplementation, together with other dietary and endogenous antioxidants, is also important.

Glutathione, an endogenously made antioxidant, represents a potent protective agent against oxidative damage in the cells. It catabolizes H_2O_2 and anions and is very effective in neutralizing peroxynitrite, a powerful form of free radicals derived from nitrogen. Therefore, increasing the intracellular levels of glutathione is essential for the protection of various components within the cells. Oral supplementation with glutathione does not significantly increase plasma levels of glutathione in humans, suggesting that this antioxidant is completely destroyed in the gastrointestinal tract. N-acetylcysteine is not destroyed in the intestinal tract, and when it enters the cells, n-acetyl is removed, and cysteine is used to make glutathione. Alpha-lipoic acid, an endogenously made antioxidant, also increases the level of glutathione in the cells. Therefore, in order to increase the level of glutathione optimally, it is necessary to use both n-acetylcysteine and alpha-lipoic acid in a multivitamin preparation for clinical studies.

Coenzyme Q10, an endogenously made antioxidant, is needed by the mitochondria to generate energy. In addition it also scavenges peroxy radicals faster than alpha-tocopherol, and like vitamin C, it can regenerate vitamin E. Therefore, the addition of coenzyme Q10 to a multivitamin preparation is valuable so as to achieve an optimal beneficial effect. In addition B vitamins that reduce homocysteine levels should be added to a multivitamin preparation, as well as vitamin D and appropriate minerals.

SUGGESTED DOSE AND
DOSE-SCHEDULE IN CLINICAL STUDIES

In clinical studies doses of a single antioxidant such as vitamin E varied from 400 IU to 1,200 IU. The doses of all ingredients in a multivitamin preparation, especially dietary and endogenous antioxidants, should be higher than the Recommended Dietary Allowances (RDA) levels, but nontoxic. Higher doses of antioxidants that inhibit oxidative stress as well as inflammation are needed. Lower doses of antioxidants may reduce oxidative stress but not chronic inflammation.

Most clinical studies to date have utilized a once-a-day dose-schedule. As we have discussed earlier, taking vitamins and antioxidants once a day creates large fluctuations of their levels in the body. This is due to the fact that the biological half-lives of vitamins and antioxidants vary markedly depending upon their lipid or water solubility. A 2-fold difference in the levels of vitamin E succinate can produce marked alterations in the expression profiles of several genes in neuroblastoma cells in culture.

The large fluctuations that this produces in the body can create genetic stress in the cells, which may compromise the effectiveness of vitamin supplementation after long-term consumption of it. Therefore, we recommend taking a multivitamin preparation twice a day in order to maintain a more constant level of vitamins and antioxidants in the body. Such a dose-schedule may improve the effectiveness of a multivitamin preparation in reducing the risk of heart disease.

Most clinical studies have utilized omega-3 fatty acids alone in order to evaluate their effectiveness in reducing the risk of heart disease. Omega-3 fatty acid supplementation has produced some beneficial effects. Therefore, in addition to consuming a preparation of multivitamins, taking omega-3 fatty acids may be valuable in reducing the risk of heart disease in an optimal manner.

A Note about Toxicity*

Antioxidants at doses higher than those that are recommended for the proposed micronutrient preparations have been consumed by the U.S. population for decades without any significant toxicity being recorded. However, they could be harmful at certain high doses for some individuals when consumed daily for a long period of time.

For example, vitamin A at doses of 10,000 IU or higher per day can cause birth defects in pregnant women, and as discussed earlier beta-carotene at doses of 50 mg or higher per day can produce bronzing of the skin that is reversible on discontinuation. Vitamin C as ascorbic acid at high doses (10 grams or higher per day) can cause diarrhea in some individuals, and vitamin E at high doses (2,000 IU or higher per day) can induce clotting defects after long-term consumption. Vitamin B6 at high doses (50 mg or higher per day) may produce peripheral neuropathy (numbness of the extremities), and selenium at doses of 400 mcg or higher per day can cause skin and liver toxicity after long-term consumption.

Coenzyme Q10 has no known toxicity; recommended daily doses are 30 to 400 mg. N-acetylcysteine at doses of 250 to 500 mg and alpha-lipoic acid at doses of 600 mg per day are utilized by humans without

---

*References listed in this section have been described in a review (Kumar et al. 2000).

toxicity. All ingredients present in the proposed micronutrient preparations (for suggested use in clinical studies) are safe and come under the category of "food supplement." Therefore, they do not require FDA approval for their use.

HOW TO RESOLVE
PRESENT CONTROVERSIES ABOUT
CLINICAL STUDIES AND THEIR EFFICACY

The inconsistent results obtained by the use of one or two dietary or endogenous antioxidants, B vitamins, and omega-3 fatty acids alone in a high-risk population suggests that such experimental designs are not sufficient to determine the effectiveness of vitamins and antioxidants in reducing the risk of heart disease in humans. The fate of individual antioxidants in a high oxidative environment also suggests that the use of a single antioxidant may be counterproductive.

Thus I suggest that a multiple micronutrient preparation containing dietary and endogenous antioxidants, the appropriate minerals and omega-3 fatty acids, together with a diet low in fat and high in fiber, and changes in lifestyle (see chapter 9 for particulars), should be included in any clinical trial that examines the concern of heart disease and its prevention. The doses of antioxidants and vitamins should be higher than the RDA (Recommended Dietary Allowances) values but not toxic.

The suggested ingredients of a multiple micronutrient supplement to be used in a clinical trial were discussed a little earlier in this chapter, but let me be more specific here. The preparation of a multiple micronutrient should contain dietary antioxidants such as vitamin A and natural mixed carotenoids (90 percent representing beta-carotene); two forms of vitamin E (d-alpha-tocopheryl acetate and d-alpha-tocopheryl succinate, also called vitamin E succinate); vitamin C (calcium ascorbate); and endogenous antioxidants such as alpha-lipoic acid; n-acetylcysteine; coenzyme Q10; L-carnitine; vitamin D; all of the B vitamins, and minerals such as selenium (selenomethionine), zinc, calcium, magnesium, and chromium picolinate.

It should be noted that both vitamin A and beta-carotene have been suggested because beta-carotene, in addition to acting as a precursor of vitamin A, performs unique functions that cannot be produced by vitamin A, and vice versa. Beta-carotene is more effective in destroying oxygen radicals than most other antioxidants. Thus, the addition of both vitamin A and beta-carotene may enhance the efficacy of a micronutrient preparation in heart-disease prevention.

The proposed micronutrient preparation contains two forms of vitamin E. Vitamin E succinate is, as we know, considered the most effective form of vitamin E because it is more soluble than alpha-tocopherol or alpha-tocopheryl acetate. It enters the cells more easily, where it is converted to alpha-tocopherol, and thus it provides intracellular (within the cell) protection against oxidative damage. It also has its own unique function as vitamin E succinate because it alters the expression of many genes in mammalian cells in culture. Therefore, in order to increase the efficacy of vitamin E, the addition of both forms of vitamin E is suggested.

Omega-3 fatty acids should be added as an additional ingredient.

This micronutrient preparation contains no herbs or herbal antioxidants. This is due to the fact that certain herbs may interact with prescription and over-the-counter drugs in an adverse manner. However, resveratrol and curcumin have produced some beneficial effects in heart disease; therefore, they can be added to a mulitple vitamin preparation.

The proposed micronutrient formulation does not contain iron, copper, or manganese because they are known to combine with vitamin C and produce excessive amounts of free radicals, which may reduce the optimal effects of the formula. In addition, in the presence of antioxidants, these trace minerals are absorbed more efficiently and may increase free forms of them in the body. As discussed earlier but bears mentioning again, increased stores of free iron or copper (wherein they are not bound to any proteins) have been associated with an increased risk of some chronic human diseases, including heart disease.

The placebo group in the proposed experimental design should not have any dietary recommendations or changes in lifestyle. Dietary and lifestyle compliances can be monitored by questionnaires, and the compliances for the micronutrient group can be monitored by measuring plasma (blood) levels of selected micronutrients every six months. This will test the effectiveness of three components together (multivitamins, omega-3 fatty acid supplements, and changes in the diet and lifestyle).

In a subgroup of the same high-risk population, the effectiveness of vitamins and antioxidants together with omega-3 fatty acids is determined by providing the placebo group with the same recommendations for changes in the diet and lifestyle as for the vitamin-omega-3 fatty acid supplement group. The results of these studies provide conclusive proof as to whether or not a vitamin-omega-3 fatty acid supplement, together with changes in diet and lifestyle, produces a more beneficial effect on reducing the risk of heart disease compared to those receiving only the vitamin-omega-3 fatty acid supplement.

One may argue that the proposed design of a clinical study is complicated because at the end of the study we may not know which particular vitamin or omega-3 fatty acid or diet and lifestyle change is responsible for a reduction in the incidence of heart disease. This argument may not be valid because the primary aim of any clinical study is to achieve success in reducing the risk of the disease. For a mechanistic study on vitamins or omega-3 fatty acids, the effects of a single antioxidant or multiple antioxidants are best studied in animal and cell-culture models.

CONCLUDING REMARKS

Despite decades of clinical trials primarily with a single dietary antioxidant in high-risk populations of developing heart disease, controversy still exists about the usefulness of antioxidant supplements. I have critically examined the results of these studies and concluded that the present trends in clinical research—using a single antioxidant to evaluate the effectiveness of vitamins and antioxidants in reducing the risk of heart disease—lack scientific rationale, and therefore have not yielded consistent beneficial effects.

I have provided potential reasons for the controversies that exist at this time in regard to this. I have also provided rationale and evidence for a shift in the design of clinical studies—from using one antioxidant alone to using a multivitamin preparation containing dietary and endogenous antioxidants, B vitamins, vitamin D, appropriate minerals, and omega-3 fatty acids, together with a diet low in fat and high in fiber.

As we have learned, the design of many studies is flawed in that they do not take into account all of the six criteria that should be part and parcel of every study undertaken. These factors include a determination of the ideal patient population; its levels of oxidative stress and chronic inflammation; number of vitamins and antioxidants (single vs. multiple) to be utilized in the study; form, type, dose, and dose-schedule of vitamins and antioxidants to be utilized in the study; primary and secondary end points of the study; and length of the study.

Specifically, traditional clinical intervention studies have utilized exogenous antioxidants but not endogenous ones; individual antioxidants or a few but not a *multiple* administration of same; varying study populations; differing clinical outcomes; and differing length of the study period. It is my view that these variables should be included in every clinical trial undertaken, and they should be standardized as much as possible in order to more accurately analyze and determine the risk of heart disease today and how we might best offset its damaging effects. Well-designed clinical studies can also measure the effectiveness of proposed supplementations in vulnerable populations. Such studies would resolve the current controversies regarding the value of vitamins and antioxidants in reducing the risk of heart disease.

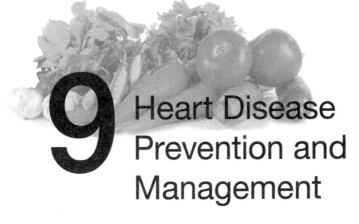

9 Heart Disease Prevention and Management

Multi-micronutrients, Diet, and Lifestyle Recommendations

In 2010 there were 981,000 cases of heart disease: a figure that is expected to rise to 1,234,000 by 2040. In 2010 there were 392,000 deaths from heart disease. This number is expected to rise to 610,000 by 2040. The financial costs to society are likewise enormous. The total direct medical cost of heart disease in 2010 was $273 billion and indirect costs were approximately $172 billion. These direct costs are projected to increase to $818 billion by 2030 and the indirect costs are expected to be in the neighborhood of $276 billion. These figures make it imperative that we develop better and additional strategies for the prevention of heart disease. This chapter describes one such strategy, which would utilize multiple micronutrients in an attempt to stem the projected increases of this debilitating disease. We include various tables to better assist the consumer in ascertaining which recommenced multi-micronutrient supplement is best for them. We then go on to discuss current findings and suggested multiple-micronutrient supplementation in combination with standard care.

TYPES OF PREVENTION STRATEGIES

Prevention strategies can be divided into two groups: primary prevention and secondary prevention. The purpose of primary prevention is to protect healthy individuals from developing heart disease. Primary prevention includes recommendations to avoid exposure to those agents that can induce one or more risk factors for developing heart disease.

The purpose of secondary prevention is to stop or slow the progression of heart disease in individuals who suffer from it. Secondary prevention strategies may involve medications such as statins (cholesterol-lowering drugs), ACE-inhibitors (ACE) and angiotensin receptor blockers (ARB; drugs like Diovan that lower blood pressure), and vitamin supplements, together with changes in diet and lifestyle.

Primary and secondary prevention strategies for individuals are implemented at the doctor's office or in the hospital. For entire populations they can be implemented at the community, state, or national level.

RECOMMENDATIONS FOR PRIMARY PREVENTION

Changes in Diet and Lifestyle

Primary prevention strategies should be adopted from childhood. These strategies include dietary and lifestyle changes, which are very important in primary prevention. A diet high in fat and rich in calories and a lifestyle marked by physical inactivity contribute to obesity, which is considered one of the major risk factors in the development of heart disease. Increased levels of oxidative stress and inflammation are found in obese individuals.

In order to reduce obesity, oxidative stress, and chronic inflammation, I recommend the daily consumption of a low-fat, high-fiber diet, with plenty of fruit (especially grapes and berries) and leafy vegetables, and avoiding an excessive intake of carbohydrates and proteins. Whenever oil is used for cooking, virgin olive oil is preferred. For non-vegetarians the consumption of fish, especially salmon twice a week and chicken and other meats—not more than four ounces per meal—is recommended. For vegetarians an increased intake of lima beans and soy/soy products is recommended. Certain spices and herbs such as turmeric, cinnamon, garlic, and ginger can be added to preparations of vegetables and meat. These spices and herbs have exhibited antioxidant and anti-inflammatory activities. It should be pointed out that herbal antioxidants, as well as standard dietary and endogenous antioxidants, produce biological effects (such as changes in gene expression, which can have a beneficial effect on diabetes), some of them not related to decreasing oxidative stress or chronic inflammation.

Recommendations that pertain to lifestyle changes include the cessation of both tobacco smoking and the chewing of tobacco, avoiding secondhand smoke, restricting one's intake of alcohol and caffeinated drinks, reducing stress (by vacationing more frequently, practicing yoga and/or mediation), and performing moderate exercise four to five times a week. Moderate exercise includes walking twenty to twenty-five minutes per day at least five days per week or using a treadmill (twenty-five minutes at a moderate speed), and weight lifting for thirty minutes three to four times a week. (The level of exercise will depend on the age of the individual.) Younger individuals can typically undertake more strenuous exercise than older people.

Changes in diet and lifestyle that reduce the risk of heart disease appear to be easy to implement but in reality are difficult to follow consistently; human behavior and habits are very difficult to change. This is supported by the fact that despite extensive educational programs about common sense changes that one can make in one's diet and lifestyle, including a cessation of cigarette smoking, the incidence of obesity has increased in the United States, and the number of people who smoke tobacco has not significantly decreased.

Micronutrient Supplements

An appropriate preparation of multiple micronutrients is important for primary prevention. This complements the effects of changes in diet and lifestyle in reducing the risk of heart disease. Micronutrients include dietary antioxidants (vitamin A, beta-carotene, vitamin C, vitamin E, and selenium), and endogenous ones (alpha-lipoic acid, the glutathione-elevating agent n-acetylcysteine or NAC, coenzyme Q10, and L-carnitine), vitamin D, B vitamins, and appropriate minerals. Omega-3 fatty acids, curcumin, and resveratrol can also be added to a multiple vitamin preparation, because they have produced some benefit in heart disease when used individually.

The doses of each of these ingredients in a micronutrient formulation will differ depending upon the age of the individual. Micronutrient formulations for various age groups (five to ten years; eleven to seventeen years, eighteen to thirty-five years, thirty-six to fifty years), with no risk factors for heart disease are presented in Tables 9.1–9.4.

For these age groups I suggest a micronutrient formulation known as BioArmor Heart (www.multimmunity.com). It is based on the original formulation of Sevak and Sevak Jr., and has been patented by the Premier Micronutrient Corporation under my purview. BioArmor has some unique properties that are not found in other multivitamin preparations currently on the market. For example, it has no iron, copper, manganese, or heavy metals (vanadium, zirconium, and molybdenum). Nor does it contain herbs or herbal antioxidants. Iron and copper are not added because they are known to interact with vitamin C and generate excessive amounts of free radicals. In addition prolonged consumption of these trace minerals in the presence of antioxidants may increase the levels of free iron or copper stores in the body because there are no significant mechanisms of excreting iron among postmenopausal women or men of all ages. Increased stores of free iron may increase the risk of some chronic human diseases, including heart disease.

Please note that in Tables 9.4, 9.5, and 9.7 the dosing amounts for certain micronutrients have not been included as they must remain proprietary.

Also please note that to some of these formulations I have made a minor modification by adding omega-3 fatty acids back into the formula, as well as natural, mixed carotenoids. The addition of omega-3 fatty acids was considered essential because of their beneficial effects noted in most clinical studies pertaining to a reduction in the progression of heart disease. The addition of carotenoids was due to a growing understanding of the significant role they play in mitigating the incidence of cardiac concerns.

TABLE 9.1. FORMULATION FOR CHILDREN (AGES 5–10)

Vitamin A (palmitate)	1,500 IU
Natural mixed carotenoids	5 mg
Vitamin C (as calcium ascorbate)	100 mg
Vitamin D$_3$ (cholecalciferol)	400 IU
Vitamin E (two forms)	50 IU d-alpha-tocopheryl acetate 25 IU d-alpha-tocopheryl acid succinate 25 IU
Vitamin B$_1$ (thiamine mononitrate)	2 mg
Vitamin B$_2$ (riboflavin)	2 mg
Niacin (as niacinamide ascorbate)	10 mg
Vitamin B$_6$ (pyridoxine HCl)	2 mg
Folate (folic acid)	400 mcg
Vitamin B$_{12}$ (as cyanocobalamin)	5 mcg
Biotin	100 mcg
Pantothenic acid (as d-calcium pantothenate)	5 mg
Calcium citrate	100 mg
Magnesium citrate	50 mg
Zinc glycinate	7.5 mg
Selenium (L-selenomethionine)	50 mcg

Total capsules per day can be taken orally, half in the morning and half in the evening.

Heavy metals were not added because prolonged consumption of them may increase stores of them in the body, given that there is no significant mechanism by which the body can excrete them. High levels of these metals are considered neurotoxic and can damage nerve cells. Herbs were not added because some herbs are known to interact adversely with prescription and non-prescription drugs.

TABLE 9.2. FORMULATION FOR ADOLESCENTS (AGES 11–17)

Vitamin A (palmitate)	2,000 IU	
Natural mixed carotenoids	5 mg	
Vitamin C (as calcium ascorbate)	250 mg	
Vitamin D$_3$ (cholecalciferol)	400 IU	
Vitamin E (two forms)	100 IU	
	d-alpha-tocopheryl acetate	50 IU
	d-alpha-tocopheryl acid succinate	50 IU
Vitamin B$_1$ (thiamine mononitrate)	2 mg	
Vitamin B$_2$ (riboflavin)	2.5 mg	
Vitamin B$_3$ (as niacinamide ascorbate)	15 mg	
Vitamin B$_6$ (pyridoxine HCl)	2.5 mg	
Folate (folic acid)	400 mcg	
Vitamin B$_{12}$ (as cyanocobalamin)	10 mcg	
Biotin	100 mcg	
Pantothenic acid (as d-calcium pantothenate)	5 mg	
Calcium citrate	125 mg	
Magnesium citrate	62.5 mg	
Zinc glycinate	7.5 mg	
Selenium (L-selenomethionine)	50 mcg	
Chromium (as chromium picolinate)	25 mcg	

Total capsules per day can be taken orally, half in the morning and half in the evening.

TABLE 9.3. FORMULATION FOR YOUNG ADULTS
(AGES 18–35)

Vitamin A (palmitate)	3,000 IU
Natural mixed carotenoids	15 mg
Vitamin C (as calcium ascorbate)	500 mg
Vitamin D₃ (cholecalciferol)	800 IU
Vitamin E (two forms)	200 IU d-alpha-tocopheryl acetate 100 IU d-alpha-tocopheryl acid succinate 100 IU
Vitamin B₁ (thiamine mononitrate)	4 mg
Vitamin B₂ (riboflavin)	5 mg
Vitamin B₃ (as niacinamide ascorbate)	30 mg
Vitamin B₆ (pyridoxine HCl)	5 mg
Folate (folic acid)	800 mcg
Vitamin B₁₂ (as cyanocobalamin)	10 mcg
Biotin	200 mcg
Pantothenic acid (as d-calcium pantothenate)	10 mg
Calcium citrate	250 mg
Magnesium citrate	125 mg
Zinc glycinate	15 mg
Selenium (L-selenomethionine)	100 mcg

Total capsules per day can be taken orally, half in the morning and half in the evening.

Most previous clinical studies in primary prevention have utilized one or two dietary antioxidants. As regards secondary prevention, most studies have utilized one or multiple dietary antioxidants. The Physicians' Health Study II was a randomized controlled trial involving 14,641 male U.S. physicians, including 754 men with a history of heart disease. In this study the effectiveness of a commercially available multivitamin

TABLE 9.4. FORMULATION FOR ADULTS (AGES 36–50) WITH NO ESTABLISHED RISK FACTORS FOR HEART DISEASE

Vitamin A (palmitate)	3,000 IU
Vitamin E (two forms)	400 IU d-alpha-tocopheryl succinate 300 IU d-alpha-tocopheryl acetate 100 IU
Vitamin C (calcium ascorbate)	1,000 mg
Vitamin D$_3$ (cholecalciferol)	800 IU
Vitamin B$_1$ (thiamine mononitrate)	4 mg
Vitamin B$_2$ (riboflavin)	5 mg
Vitamin B$_3$ (niacinamide ascorbate)	30 mg
Vitamin B$_6$ (pyridoxine HCl)	5 mg
Folate (folic acid)	800 mcg
Vitamin B$_{12}$ (as cyanocobalamin)	10 mcg
Biotin	200 mcg
Pantothenic acid (d-calcium pantothenate)	10 mg
Calcium citrate	250 mg
Magnesium citrate	125 mg
Zinc glycinate	15 mg
Selenium (Seleno-L-methionine, also called L-selenomethionine)	100 mcg
Chromium (as picolinate)	50 mcg
Total amounts of antioxidants listed below is 1,065 mg.	
Alpha-lipoic acid	proprietary amount
Coenzyme Q10	proprietary amount
Curcumin	proprietary amount
L-carnitine	proprietary amount
n-acetylcysteine (NAC)	proprietary amount
Natural mixed carotenoids	proprietary amount
Omega-3 fatty acids	proprietary amount
Resveratrol	proprietary amount

Total capsules per day can be taken orally, half in the morning and half in the evening.

preparation (Centrum Silver) was evaluated in order to ascertain its ability to reduce the risk of major heart-disease events. These primary events included nonfatal myocardial infarction, nonfatal stroke, and death from heart disease, and secondary heart disease events such as myocardial infarction and stroke individually. The median follow-up period was 11.2 years, at which time the results were determined (Sesso et al. 2012).

The finding was that supplementation with this preparation of multivitamins did not reduce major cardiac events. The exact reason for this is unknown; however, I speculate that it may have been because this preparation of multivitamins did not contain endogenous antioxidants such as alpha-lipoic acid, coenzyme Q10, and L-carnitine. The multivitamins used in this study did not contain n-acetylcysteine, nor did they contain omega-3 fatty acids, which appear to be useful in reducing the risk of heart disease.

The results of all of the primary and secondary prevention clinical studies yielded inconsistent results that varied from some transient beneficial effects, to no effects, to harmful effects. The possible reasons for these inconsistent results include the following:

1. The use of only one or two dietary or endogenous antioxidants
2. The use of multivitamins containing only dietary antioxidants
3. The failure to use a micronutrient preparation containing multiple dietary antioxidants (vitamin A, B vitamins, beta-carotene, vitamin C, vitamin D, vitamin E, and the mineral selenium) and endogenous antioxidants (n-acetylcysteine, alpha-lipoic acid, coenzyme Q10, and L-carnitine)
4. The use of omega-3 fatty acids, or low-dose aspirin alone, rather than in combination with a micronutrient preparation as described above
5. The failure to utilize a dose-schedule of twice a day (morning and evening) to achieve a more constant level of micronutrients in the body

RECOMMENDATIONS
FOR SECONDARY PREVENTION

Generally, individuals age fifty or older develop one or more risk factors for heart disease. However, in some people heart disease may develop earlier. Risk factors common to both groups include high levels of total cholesterol, LDL cholesterol, and triglycerides; low levels of HDL cholesterol; increased plasma levels of C-reactive protein and homocysteine; and increased levels of markers of oxidative stress and chronic inflammation.

Secondary prevention is recommended for those individuals who have not had any major heart disease events such as heart attack, atrial or ventricular fibrillation, or stroke, but who have developed one or more risk factors for heart disease as described above. Secondary prevention must include changes in diet and lifestyle, a micronutrient preparation containing multiple dietary and endogenous antioxidants, standard medications for lowering cholesterol and blood pressure (statins and ACE/ARB with or without hydrochlorothiazide [HCT]), and low-dose aspirin.

Changes in Diet and Lifestyle

Dietary and lifestyle changes are very important in secondary prevention; they are the same as those described for primary prevention (see pages 145–46).

Low-Dose Aspirin

Low-dose aspirin (acetylsalicylic acid) at a dose of 81 mg per day is commonly recommended for reducing the risk and progression of heart disease because it prevents platelet aggregation by reducing the production of prostaglandins. Aspirin has been shown to reduce major cardiac or cerebral events by 25 percent (Macchi et al. 2006).

However, it has been reported that about 5 to 12 percent of patients with heart disease develop resistance to aspirin (Cotter et al. 2004; Gum et al. 2003).

Another study estimated that 8 to 45 percent of patients taking aspirin develop aspirin resistance (Patel and Moonis 2007).

Furthermore, about 24 percent of patients taking aspirin displayed a reduced response with respect to platelet aggregation (they are referred to as semi-responders) (Gum et al. 2001).

This has required physicians to increase aspirin doses in those patients who develop aspirin resistance or become semi-responders. Given that high doses of aspirin may cause internal bleeding, this increase was done until the toxic limit was reached. However, aspirin resistance continued to be present in some cases despite increased aspirin doses. It has been reported that the risk of major cardiac events may increase by about 3-fold in aspirin-resistant patients (Gum et al. 2003). Therefore, resolving the issue of aspirin resistance has become a new challenge for researchers in cardiology.

Although the mechanisms of aspirin resistance are not known, we suggest that the addition of multiple antioxidants may enhance the effectiveness of low-dose aspirin in reducing platelet aggregation. This is substantiated by the fact that vitamin E in combination with aspirin is more effective in inhibiting cyclooxygenase-1 (COX-1) enzyme activity than the individual agent (Abate et al. 2000). This enzyme is responsible for the production of prostaglandins, which cause platelet aggregation. Thus, supplementation with multiple dietary and endogenous antioxidants may prolong the effectiveness of aspirin among semi-responders as well as in patients who develop a total resistance to aspirin. This should be tested in a well-designed clinical study.

Micronutrient Supplements

An appropriate preparation of micronutrients containing dietary and endogenous antioxidants is, as noted above, important for secondary prevention, but it is not currently being recommended by state or national agencies. And although the U.S. Preventive Service Task Force recommends multivitamin supplements to reduce the risk of cancer and heart disease (U.S. Preventive Service Task Force 2003; Riley and Stouffer 2002), these recommendations do not provide guidelines with respect to the type of micronutrients that should be included in them and the micronutrients that should be excluded. The doses and dose-schedule are also not articulated.

The BioArmor formula (based on the original formulation of Sevak and Sevak Jr.), mentioned earlier, addresses these overlooked concerns. As stated previously it has been patented by the Premier Micronutrient Corporation under my purview. Its formulation is recommended to those individuals who are fifty-one years of age or older, with one or more risk factors for heart disease, but who have had no major cardiac events such as nonfatal myocardial infarction (MI), or nonfatal stroke. This formula is articulated in Table 9.5 on page 156.

The unique features of this formulation are the same described in the section on primary prevention, found on pages 147–48, so I will not repeat them here.

Standard Medications

In addition to diet and lifestyle changes, micronutrient supplements, and low-dose aspirin, gold standard medications are also recommended. These include statins for lowering cholesterol, ACE/ARB for lowering blood pressure, and low-dose aspirin for reducing inflammation and platelet aggregation.

Increased oxidative stress and chronic inflammation continue to occur during treatment with cholesterol-lowering drugs in high-risk populations. This is evidenced by the fact that the smoking of tobacco increased the risk of morbidity and mortality among heavy smokers, despite treatment with standard medications that are known to reduce cardiovascular disease (Dagenais et al. 2005). Nevertheless, treatment with cholesterol-lowering medications, as well as medications that lower blood pressure, should continue. The doses and dose-schedules of these drugs should be determined by a primary care doctor or cardiologist.

TABLE 9.5. FORMULATION FOR ADULTS WHO HAVE ONE OR MORE RISK FACTORS BUT NO MAJOR CARDIAC EVENTS

Vitamin A (palmitate)	3,000 IU
Vitamin E (two forms)	400 IU d-alpha-tocopheryl succinate 300 IU d-alpha-tocopheryl acetate 100 IU
Vitamin C (calcium ascorbate)	1,500 mg
Vitamin D$_3$ (cholecalciferol)	800 IU
Vitamin B$_1$ (thiamine mononitrate)	4 mg
Vitamin B$_2$ (riboflavin)	5 mg
Vitamin B$_3$ (niacinamide ascorbate)	30 mg
Vitamin B$_6$ (pyridoxine HCl)	5 mg
Folate (folic acid)	800 mcg
Vitamin B$_{12}$ (cyanocobalamin)	10 mcg
Biotin	200 mcg
Pantothenic acid (d-calcium pantothenate)	10 mg
Calcium citrate	250 mg
Magnesium citrate	125 mg
Zinc glycinate	15 mg
Selenium (Seleno-L-methionine, also called L-selenomethionine)	100 mcg
Chromium (as chromium picolinate)	50 mcg
Total amount of antioxidants listed below is 1,840 mg.	
Alpha-lipoic acid	proprietary amount
Coenzyme Q10	proprietary amount
Curcumin	proprietary amount
L-carnitine	proprietary amount
n-acetylcysteine (NAC)	proprietary amount
Natural mixed carotenoids	proprietary amount
Omega-3 fatty acids	proprietary amount
Resveratrol	proprietary amount

Total capsules per day can be taken orally, half in the morning and half in the evening.

RECOMMENDATIONS FOR THOSE WITH A FAMILY HISTORY OF HEART DISEASE

Individuals with a family history (genetic basis) of heart disease have an increased risk of developing heart disease at an earlier age compared to those without a family history of the same. It is often believed that the genetic basis of heart disease cannot be prevented or delayed. Therefore, individuals with a family history of it often wait until its risk factors and/or disease symptoms begin to appear before undertaking standard prevention and treatment regimens.

Recent laboratory experiments on the genetic basis of another disease (cancer) show that it may be possible to prevent or at least delay the onset of the genetic basis of heart disease. The gene HOP (TUM-1) is essential for the development of *Drosophila melanogaster* (fruit flies). A mutation in this gene markedly increases the risk of developing a leukemia-like tumor in female flies. (This is an unpublished observation from work conducted in collaboration with Dr. Bhattacharya et al. of NASA.)

Proton radiation is a powerful cancer-causing agent. Whole-body irradiation of these flies with proton radiation dramatically increased the incidence of cancer, compared to unirradiated flies. The question arose as to whether or not antioxidants can influence the incidence of cancer, which has a specific gene defect. To test this possibility, a mixture of multiple dietary and endogenous antioxidants was fed to these flies seven days before proton irradiation, and was then continued throughout the experimental period. The results showed that antioxidant treatment before and after irradiation totally blocked the formation of proton radiation–induced cancer in fruit flies.

This finding on fruit flies is of particular interest because to my knowledge this is the first demonstration in which it has been shown that the genetic basis of a disease can be prevented by antioxidant treatment. It is not known whether antioxidants can prevent the onset of heart disease in those individuals who have a hereditary genetic basis (family history) of it. However, the results on fruit flies and cancer have raised the possibility that this may indeed be possible.

Those individuals with a family history of heart disease should consider adopting the proposed recommendations made for primary prevention found on pages 145–50. The recommendations should be followed from childhood on. Additionally, the secondary prevention strategies, found on pages 153–56 should be adopted as well.

RECOMMENDATIONS IN COMBINATION WITH STANDARD CARE

High-risk heart-disease patients with high blood pressure and/or stenosis, or who have experienced at least one major cardiac event such as myocardial infarction, bypass surgery, or stroke, are considered suitable for a study that evaluates the role of micronutrients, as well as diet and lifestyle changes, in combination with standard care for the treatment of heart disease. Standard care is typically understood to mean the administration by cardiologists of conventional drugs and therapies designed to help a patient heal. Currently used standard therapies include statins, angiotensin-converting enzyme inhibitors, beta-blockers, anti-inflammatory drugs, and surgical interventions (angioplasty, bypass surgery, heart transplants), followed by various forms of rehabilitation therapy, depending on the type of surgery one has had.

Since increased oxidative stress and chronic inflammation play a contributing role in the progression of major heart disease events, supplementation with antioxidants that reduce oxidative stress and chronic inflammation appears to be a wise choice of treatment protocol in this context. However, as we know, only a *few* studies with individual antioxidants and omega-3 fatty acids have been performed on this issue. *No* studies have been performed to evaluate the efficacy of a micronutrient preparation containing multiple dietary and endogenous antioxidants, B vitamins, vitamin D, omega-3 fatty acids, and certain minerals in combination with standard care.

This section describes the results of studies that have been performed on the effects of antioxidants alone or in combination with standard care for the treatment of heart disease. In addition, it proposes the scientific basis of a micronutrient formulation that can be used in combination with it.

The Effect of Coenzyme Q10 Alone

Coenzyme Q10 appears to be significant in the treatment of heart failure. In a clinical study involving eleven patients who were candidates for a heart transplant received coenzyme Q10 orally. All patients showed improvement and some of them required no standard medication and no limitation in lifestyle (Folkers et al. 1992).

In a clinical study involving seventeen patients with a congestive heart failure, the effectiveness of coenzyme Q10 in improving the symptoms of this disease was tested. After four months of coenzyme Q10 supplementation, most symptoms, as noted by congestive heart failure score, cardiac output, stroke volume index, and systolic blood pressure, improved (Sacher et al. 1997).

In a clinical study involving forty-three patients who had 50 percent stenosis (the narrowing of a coronary artery) or who had undergone angioplasty, it was demonstrated that after twelve weeks of oral administration with coenzyme Q10 at a dose of 150 mg per day, oxidative stress decreased and the antioxidant enzymes catalase and superoxide dismutase increased, compared to the placebo group (Lee et al. 2012a).

Using the same population of forty patients, coenzyme Q10 treatment at a dose of 150 mg per day decreased markers of pro-inflammatory cytokines (interleukin-6 and C-reactive protein) and oxidative stress, but it did not decrease homocysteine levels (Lee et al. 2012b).

Coenzyme Q10 in combination with standard therapy improved the function of damaged cardiac muscle associated with congestive heart failure (Judy et al. 1991) and idiopathic dilated cardiomyopathy (a form of heart disease in which the heart chambers are enlarged) (Langsjoen et al. 1990).

The Effect of Vitamin E Alone

In a clinical study involving ninety patients with heart disease, the effectiveness of natural vitamin E alone on the incidence of heart disease events was tested. The results showed that vitamin E supplementation reduced the levels of markers of oxidative stress and inflammation, but did not change the thickness of the wall of the carotid artery or events associated with heart disease when compared to those who received placebo pills (Devaraj et al. 2007).

One clinical study featured 8,415 patients who had already experienced one myocardial infarction but had no congestive heart failure at the beginning of the trial. The results showed that supplementation with vitamin E alone increased the risk of congestive heart failure by about 20 percent, which was not considered significant because of a large variation in the values of congestive heart failure as measured from one patient to another. However, vitamin E supplementation increased the risk of congestive heart failure by about 50 percent in those patients who had left ventricle dysfunction. This was found to be significant (Marchioli et al. 2006).

These studies were not confirmed in a recent clinical study referred to as the Women's Health Study. In this study which involved 39,815 healthy women of at least forty-five years of age, the effectiveness of vitamin E on heart failure was tested; it was administered at an oral dose of 600 IU every other day. The results showed that vitamin E supplementation did not increase the risk of heart failure. The possibility of a beneficial effect on diastolic heart failure was suggested, but was not considered to be statistically significant by the authors (Chae et al. 2012).

Another study using 156 men with previous coronary bypass surgery who were receiving a cholesterol-lowering drug combination (colestipol-niacin) alone or in combination with 100 IU of vitamin E per day showed that the group that had been treated with vitamin E showed less progression of the narrowing of their coronary arteries compared to cholesterol-lowering drugs alone during a four-year trial period (Hodis et al. 1995) (Table 9.6).

**TABLE 9.6. THE EFFECT OF ANTIOXIDANTS IN COMBINATION
WITH CHOLESTEROL-LOWERING DRUGS IN HIGH-RISK PATIENTS
WITH HEART DISEASE ON STANDARD CARE**

Study	No. of patients	Antioxidants + cholesterol-lowering drugs	Clinical outcome	Follow-up	Results
a. CLAS	156	Colestipol + niacin + Vit. E 100 IC per day or higher	Stenosis	2 years	Reduced
b.	126	Coenzyme Q10 33.3 mg (thrice a day)	Cardiac muscle function	6 years	Improved

Key:
CLAS (Cholesterol-Lowering Atherosclerosis Study)
a. The patients were men 40 to 59 years of age who had undergone previous coronary artery bypass graft surgery
b. Idiopathic dilated cardiomyopathy
All vitamins were administered in a once-a-day dose-schedule unless otherwise specified.
Total capsules per day can be taken orally, half in the morning and half in the evening.

The Effect of Vitamin C Alone

In a rat model of ventricular fibrillation and electric shock, the effect of vitamin C (ascorbic acid) administered intravenously (100 mg per kilogram of body weight) on damage to the heart during cardiopulmonary resuscitation (CPR), was studied. The results showed that vitamin C administered at the start of CPR reduced oxidative stress. This was indicated by a reduction in malondialdehyde, (a marker of oxidative stress). Vitamin C also reduced damage to heart muscle cells and mitochondria, facilitated CPR, and improve outcomes following ventricular fibrillation and electric shock (Tsai et al. 2011). No such study has been performed on humans.

Microcirculation is impaired during ischemia-reperfusion in patients undergoing elective coronary angioplasty. In a clinical study involving fifty-six patients undergoing coronary angioplasty, the effectiveness of 1 gram of vitamin C on microcirculation during reperfusion was determined. The vitamin C was administered intravenously at the rate of 16.6 mg per minute for a period of one hour. The results showed that the vitamin C improved microcirculation compared to that found in the placebo group (Basili et al. 2010).

The Effect of Vitamin C and Vitamin E

Patients who have received heart transplants have an increased risk of developing coronary atherosclerosis, which reduces one's chances of long-term survival and is a major cause of death. Increased oxidative stress has been implicated in the development of coronary atherosclerosis in patients with heart transplants. Treatment with a mixture of vitamins C and E reduced the progression of coronary atherosclerosis in these patients (Liu and Meydani 2002).

In another clinical study involving forty patients with heart transplants, supplementation with vitamin C 500 mg twice a day and vitamin E 400 IU twice a day for one year reduced atherosclerosis in patients with normal and/or abnormal endothelial function. However, the magnitude of beneficial effects was larger in patients with endothelial dysfunction (Behrendt et al. 2006).

About 30 percent of patients developed atrial fibrillation after heart surgery. Increased oxidative stress is thought to be one of the contributing factors in the development of atrial fibrillation. Prior treatment with vitamins C and E reduced the incidence of atrial fibrillation in these patients (Harling et al. 2011).

The Effect of N-acetylcysteine Alone

A review of eight clinical trials showed that supplementation with n-acetylcysteine before heart surgery reduced the incidence of atrial fibrillation after surgery (Gu et al. 2012). Although short-term treatment benefits were observed in some clinical studies, we do not recommend one or two antioxidants for long-term benefit. This is due to the fact that individual antioxidants in high-risk populations are oxidized due to the high internal oxidative environments of these patients.

The Effect of Omega-3 Fatty Acids Alone

As we know atrial fibrillation is a common complication following coronary artery bypass surgery. A review of several studies suggested that supplementation with omega-3 fatty acids administered *orally* reduced the incidence of post-heart-surgery atrial fibrillation. It also reduced the incidence of sudden death in survivors of heart attack (Lombardi and Terranova 2007).

A preoperative *intravenous* infusion of omega-3 fatty acids also reduced the incidence of atrial fibrillation after heart surgery, and shortened stays in the intensive care unit and in the hospital (Calo et al. 2005; Heidt et al. 2009).

It has been reported that certain heart disease patients who exhibit angina (chest pain) and some individuals with a history of ventricular arrhythmia (abnormal heart rhythm) may not derive any benefit from supplementation with omega-3 fatty acids (Jenkins et al. 2008).

A review of published studies on the effects of omega-3 fatty acids on the incidence of recurrent ventricular arrhythmia in patients with an implantable cardioverter defibrillator (ICD) showed that these fatty acids did not provide any protection against recurrent ventricular arrhythmia (Brouwer et al. 2009).

However, in patients with diabetes who had previous myocardial infarction, supplementation with omega-3 fatty acids reduced the incidence of ventricular arrhythmia and fatal myocardial infarction (Kromhout et al. 2011).

The administration of omega-3 fatty acids but not of a statin (Rosuvastatin) significantly reduced death and admission to the hospital for symptoms associated with heart disease (Marchioli et al. 2009).

PROPOSED RECOMMENDATIONS OF MICRONUTRIENTS, DIET, AND LIFESTYLE IN COMBINATION WITH STANDARD CARE

In order to produce an optimal benefit in reducing the progression of various forms of heart disease, I propose a formulation of micronutrients and changes in diet and lifestyle in combination with standard care.

Micronutrient Formulation Recommendations

Increased oxidative stress and pro-inflammatory cytokines play a leading role in the progression of various forms of heart disease. Therefore, supplementation with a micronutrient preparation containing multiple dietary and endogenous antioxidants appears to be one of the most logical choices for reducing the progression of disease before or after surgical intervention. Indeed, the results obtained from the use of one or two antioxidants showed some beneficial effects in patients suffering from different forms of heart disease.

The BioArmor Heart formulation that I have developed (www .multimmunity.com) is recommended for those individuals who have had one or more major cardiac events such as angioplasty, nonfatal myocardial infarction, or nonfatal stroke.

The rationale for using multiple micronutrients and appropriate minerals as well as the uniqueness of this formulation, dose and dose-schedule, has been described in chapter 8. Except for increased doses of vitamin E, coenzyme Q10, L-carnitine, alpha-lipoic acid, and coenzyme Q10, the formulation of this micronutrient preparation is similar to that recommended for the secondary prevention of heart disease as found in chapter 9. Except for one clinical study that has tested the effectiveness of this formulation minus omega-3 fatty acids in primary prevention (chapter 9), no clinical study has been performed with the proposed micronutrient formulation in combination with standard therapy in the management of various forms of heart disease. Such studies should be initiated.

TABLE 9.7. FORMULATION FOR ADULTS WHO HAVE HAD ONE OR MORE MAJOR CARDIAC EVENTS

Vitamin A (palmitate)	3,000 IU
Natural Vitamin E (two forms)	600 IU d-alpha-tocopheryl succinate 500 IU d-alpha-tocopheryl acetate 100 IU
Vitamin C (calcium ascorbate)	1,500 mg
Vitamin D$_3$ (cholecalciferol)	400 IU
Vitamin B$_1$ (thiamine mononitrate)	4 mg
Vitamin B$_2$ (riboflavin)	5 mg
Vitamin B$_3$ (niacinamide ascorbate)	30 mg
Vitamin B$_6$ (pyridoxine hydrochloride)	5 mg
Folate (folic acid)	800 mcg
Vitamin B$_{12}$ (cyanocobalamin)	10 mcg
Biotin	200 mcg
Pantothenic acid (d-calcium pantothenate)	10 mg
Calcium citrate	250 mg
Magnesium citrate	125 mg
Zinc glycinate	15 mg
Selenium (seleno-L-methionine, also called L-selenomethionine)	100 mcg
Chromium (as chromium picolinate)	50 mcg
Total amounts of antioxidants listed below is 2,025 mg.	
Alpha-lipoic acid	proprietary amount
Coenzyme Q10	proprietary amount
Curcurmin	proprietary amount
L-carnitine	proprietary amount
n-acetylcysteine (NAC)	proprietary amount
Natural mixed carotenoids	proprietary amount
Omega-3 fatty acids	proprietary amount
Resveratrol	proprietary amount

Total capsules per day can be taken orally, half in the morning and half in the evening.

Diet and Lifestyle Recommendations

These recommendations are the same as those described for primary prevention on pages 145–46. Cardiologists have no objection to suggesting the proposed recommendations regarding diet and lifestyle changes to their patients.

WHAT TO EXPECT FROM
THE PROPOSED RECOMMENDATIONS

It is expected that the addition of a preparation of micronutrients and changes in diet and lifestyle to the regimen of standard care may improve the effectiveness of standard therapy and may even reduce some potentially harmful effects of drugs that are used in therapy. For example, statins, which decrease cholesterol levels, also inhibit the formation of coenzyme Q10 due to the fact that this antioxidant is in the same pathway that's used for cholesterol formation. (Coenzyme Q10 is needed for energy production by the mitochondria.) Another example involves anti-inflammatory drugs, which may be used in the treatment of heart disease. These drugs can cause bleeding and other harmful side effects. Since antioxidants may enhance the effectiveness of anti-inflammatory drugs in reducing platelet aggregation, lower doses of anti-inflammatory drugs, if used in combination with antioxidants, may be needed.

CONCLUDING REMARKS

Despite the current preventive recommendations regarding changes in diet and lifestyle to reduce the risk of heart disease, more people die of heart disease and its related complications than from any other illness or condition. Thus we know that the current guidelines for prevention are not optimal, underscoring the need to develop new solutions to this pressing concern. I have therefore proposed recommendations for both the primary and secondary prevention of heart disease, which include supplementation with a specific multiple micronutrient; it is unlike any other supplement found on the market today.

This micronutrient supplementation that I recommend is one that I have developed based on a thorough analysis of the science of the separate vitamins, antioxidants, and minerals that should be taken together, in specified doses and dose-schedules, to minimize the risk of developing one or more cardiac conditions. It can also be incorporated into a therapeutic protocol for those persons receiving standard care in connection with the complications of heart disease.

Clinical studies to test the effectiveness of the aforementioned recommendations should be initiated. In the meantime those suffering from heart disease should consider adopting them following a consultation with their cardiologist.

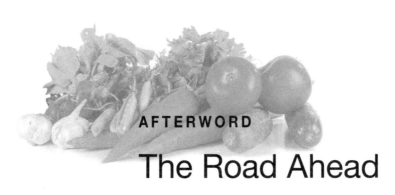

The Road Ahead

Our primary aim in writing this book is to help those individuals who either have complications of heart disease, or are at risk of developing heart disease. As we have discussed herein, some of the risk factors for developing heart disease can be acted upon, and we encourage those individuals who are at risk to take the necessary steps to mitigate its onset or its presenting symptoms. Factors that can be acted upon include physical inactivity—which may lead to a state of being overweight or obese—high blood pressure, high LDL cholesterol, the smoking of tobacco, drug abuse, increased oxidative stress, chronic inflammation, an overabundance of fat and salt in the diet, and elevated homocysteine levels—as well as an elevated production of free radicals in the body.

Our particular area of interest is the role of vitamins and antioxidants in reducing the risk of heart disease. As we have learned, physicians and cardiologists may recommend changes in diet and lifestyle to their patients to help them with their cardiac concerns, but they don't typically recommend the inclusion of a variety of vitamins and antioxidants on a regular basis. However, given that increased oxidative stress, chronic inflammation, and elevated homocysteine levels are major contributing factors to heart disease, and that vitamins and antioxidants may be extremely helpful in reducing these three conditions simultaneously—which has the potential to be very therapeutic but is not an option in terms of current treatment protocols—more research on this particular area of inquiry should be made a priority.

Regarding studies done to date, the effect of a single antioxidant on risk factors for heart disease have been performed in cell culture and with animals, with the results being that consistent beneficial effects in reducing the risk of heart disease were achieved. However, most human epidemiological and clinical intervention studies pertaining to this line of research have used only one or two dietary antioxidants. Furthermore, these studies involving the effects of individual dietary antioxidants such as vitamin E, beta-carotene, resveratrol, and omega-3 fatty acids as well as B vitamins alone on populations at high risk of developing heart disease have produced inconsistent results. These results ranged from some beneficial effects, to no effects, to harmful effects. Harmful effects may in part have occurred due to the fact that these high-risk populations have a correspondingly high oxidative internal environment, which is capable of changing a solitary antioxidant into a damaging prooxidant. It is noteworthy that a formula containing many different antioxidants serves to neutralize this damaging effect.

In terms of the inconsistent results obtained in human studies, part of the problem is that these human intervention studies are not standardized as to evaluation criteria. Currently, all of the criteria that should be included in any given study typically are not. Factors that should routinely be included in each and every study are a quantification of the ideal patient population; the degree of inherent oxidative stress and chronic inflammation in that patient population; the number of vitamins and antioxidants (single vs. multiple) to be used in the study; form, type, dose, and dose-schedule of vitamins and antioxidants to be used in the study; primary and secondary end points of study; and length of study. (Factors that are often ignored or omitted include the levels of oxidative stress and chronic inflammation present in the study population; a consideration of the number of vitamins and antioxidants to be used in the study; and a consideration of the form, type, dose, and dose-schedule of vitamins and antioxidants to be used in the study.)

Until such time that all studies are standardized in terms of these essential variables, we will continue to arrive at inconsistent results, thereby obviating the efforts of *all* of the research done on the topic.

Above I have spoken to the point that the human studies done to date have primarily included only one or two antioxidants. It is my belief that many of the current problems associated with heart disease would be mitigated by the ingestion of a multi-micronutrient supplement containing numerous vitamins and antioxidants in combinations and amounts that have been derived from exhaustive scientific analysis. (This particular thrust continues to be my current field of interest and inquiry.)

To test this and other similar end points, a pilot study was undertaken on a patient population at very high risk for manifesting cardiac issues. This high-risk population consisted of U.S. firefighters, given that they typically experience a relatively high number of heart attacks on the job. The period of study was one year and the supplement they were administered was the BioArmor Heart Formula, from the Premier Micronutrient Corporation, developed under my aegis (www .multimmunity.com). The results of this study were independently evaluated by Jeff Boone, M.D., a prominent preventive cardiologist.

The results of this study revealed a progressive decrease in LDL cholesterol and an increase in HDL cholesterol in the study population. Additionally, and perhaps more significantly, the width of the firefighters' coronary artery wall (IMT) was reduced when compared to the value observed before vitamin supplementation. (Increased IMT causes the coronary artery to narrow, potentially causing a reduction of blood that reaches the heart.) To the best of my understanding, there are no drugs on the market today that can or have achieved this same success with respect to reducing coronary IMT.

More studies like this one are needed to turn the growing tide around for, as we know, heart disease is the leading cause of death in the United States, and stroke is number four. The financial toll of heart disease and its complications on society are enormous. These costs are rising all the time, and by the year 2030 they are projected to be in the neighborhood of over 800 billion dollars.

As noted above, although it is the case that cardiologists and physicians do not recommend antioxidant and vitamin supplements to those at risk of developing heart disease or those individuals suffering from it, the U.S. Prevention Service Task Force does recommend multiple vitamin supplements to reduce the risk of heart disease. But they do not provide clear guidelines regarding the types of vitamins, antioxidants, and minerals that should be included, nor do they articulate specific dosing recommendations or dose-schedules. The RDAs/DRIs for vitamins and antioxidants have likewise been established, but these guidelines only allow for normal growth and development, and do not specifically target disease prevention as an end point. Although these current guidelines combined may provide a constructive *framework* of guidance, they clearly are not optimal. This underscores the need to develop new and better guidelines and recommendations that will successfully combat the age-old problem of heart disease.

I believe that if people at risk for developing heart disease, or those who currently suffer from its complications, follow the recommendations contained in this book, we would go a long way toward reducing the prevalence and incidence of heart disease in America today.

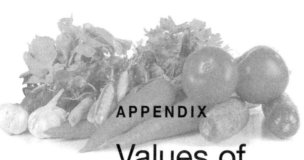

Values of Recommended Dietary Allowances (RDA)/ Dietary Reference Intakes (DRI)

Note to the Reader: All of the information contained in this appendix, including the tables, is from my book *Fighting Cancer with Vitamins and Antioxidants,* coauthored with my son K. C. Prasad, M.S., M.D., published by Healing Arts Press in 2011.

■ ■ ■

Sufficient changes in nutritional guidelines have occurred since World War II due to our increased knowledge of nutrition and health. The nutritional guidelines referred to as Recommended Dietary Allowances (RDAs) were first established in 1941. The Food and Nutrition Board of the United States subsequently revise these guidelines every five to ten years.

RDA (DRI)

RDA refers to the value of the daily dietary intake level of a nutrient considered sufficient to meet the requirements of 97 to 98 percent of healthy individuals of different ages and genders. Because of the rapid growth of research on the role of nutrients in human health, the Food and Nutrition Board of the Institute of Medicine (IOM) of the United States in collaboration with Health Canada updated the values of RDAs and renamed them Dietary Reference Intakes (DRIs) in 1998. Since then DRI values are used by both the United States and Canada. The DRI values of selected nutrients are listed in Tables A.1 to A.21. The DRI values are not currently used in nutrition labeling; the RDA values of nutrients continue to be used for this purpose. The DRI values for carotenoids, alpha-lipoic acid, n-acetylcysteine, coenzyme Q10, and L-carnitine have not been determined.

ADEQUATE INTAKE (AI)

AI refers to the value of a nutrient for which no RDA has been established, but the value established may be sufficient for everyone in the demographic group.

TOLERABLE UPPER INTAKE LEVEL (UL)

The tolerable upper intake level is the maximum level of daily nutrient intake that is likely to pose no risk of adverse health effects. The UL value represents total intake of a nutrient from food, water, and supplements.

RELATIONSHIP BETWEEN RECOMMENDED DIETARY ALLOWANCES VALUES AND OPTIMAL HEALTH

RDA values of nutrients are expected to be adequate for individuals for normal growth and survival; however, the values of micronutrients needed for prevention or improved management of human diseases are not known at this time. The data on doses obtained from the use of a single micronutrient in the prevention or treatment of human heart disease should not be extrapolated to the doses of the same micronutrient present in a multiple micronutrient preparation.

RDA/DRI values of micronutrients are sufficient for normal growth and survival, but they are not adequate for prevention or improved treatment of human diseases. In order to evaluate the dosage of micronutrients in any multivitamin preparation for the prevention or improved treatment of heart disease, it is essential to have sufficient knowledge of the RDA values of the micronutrients as found in the next section of this book.

TABLE A.1. DIETARY REFERENCE INTAKES (DRI) OF ANTIOXIDANT VITAMIN A

Age	RDA/AI*	UL
	µg/d (IU/d)	µg/d (IU/d)
Infants		
0–6 mo	400 (1,200 IU)*	600 (1,800 IU)
7–12 mo	500 (1,500 IU)*	600 (1,800 IU)
Children		
1–3 y	300 (900 IU)	600 (1,800 IU)
4–8 y	400 (1,200 IU)	900 (2,700 IU)
Males		
9–13 y	600 (1,800 IU)	1,700 (5,100 IU)
14–18 y	900 (2,700 IU)	2,800 (8,400 IU)
19 y and up	900 (2,700 IU)	3,000 (9,000 IU)
Females		
9–13 y	600 (1,800 IU)	1,700 (5,100 IU)
14–18 y	700 (2,100 IU)	2,800 (8,400 IU)
19 y and up	700 (2,100 IU)	3,000 (9,000 IU)
Pregnancy		
under 18 y	750 (2,250 IU)	2,800 (8,400 IU)
19–50 y	770 (2,310 IU)	3,000 (9,000 IU)
Lactation		
under 18 y	1,200 (3,600 IU)	2,800 (8,400 IU)
19–50 y	1,300 (3,900 IU)	3,000 (9,000 IU)

1 µg of retinol equals 1 µg of RAE (retinol activity equivalent); 1 IU of retinol equals 0.3 µg of retinol; and 2 µg of beta-carotene equals 1 µg of retinol.

RDA = Recommended Dietary Allowances
*AI = Adequate Intake
UL = Tolerable Upper Intake Value
µg = microgram; d = day

The values are adapted and summarized from the table of the Dietary Reference Intakes (DRI) published by www.nap.edu. (Search on "Food and Nutrition" and you will find information about DRI.)

TABLE A.2. DIETARY REFERENCE
INTAKES (DRI) OF ANTIOXIDANT VITAMIN C

Age	RDA/AI*	UL
	mg/d	mg/d
Infants		
0–6 mo	40*	ND
7–12 mo	50*	ND
Children		
1–3 y	15	400
4–8 y	25	650
Males		
9–13 y	45	1,200
14–18 y	75	1,800
19 y and up	90	2,000
Females		
9–13 y	45	1,200
14–18 y	65	1,800
19 y and up	75	2,000

RDA = Recommended Dietary Allowances
*AI = Adequate Intake
UL = Tolerable Upper Intake Value
µg = microgram; d = day

The values are adapted and summarized from the table of the Dietary Reference Intakes (DRI) published by www.nap.edu.

TABLE A.3. DIETARY REFERENCE
INTAKES (DRI) OF ANTIOXIDANT VITAMIN E

Age	RDA/AI*	UL
	mg/d (IU/d)	mg/d (IU/d)
Infants		
0–6 mo	4 (6 IU)*	ND
7–12 mo	5 (7.5 IU)*	ND
Children		
1–3 y	6 (9 IU)	200 (30 IU)
4–8 y	7 (10.6 IU)	300 (45 IU)
Males		
9–13 y	11 (16.7 IU)	600 (90 IU)
14–18 y	15 (22.8 IU)	800 (120 IU)
19 y and up	15 (22.8 IU)	1,000 (150 IU)
Females		
9–13 y	11 (16.7 IU)	600 (90 IU)
14–18 y	15 (22.8 IU)	800 (120 IU)
19 y and up	15 (22.8 IU)	1,000 (150 IU)
Pregnancy		
under 18 y	15 (22.8 IU)	800 (120 IU)
19–50 y	15 (22.8 IU)	1,000 (150 IU)
Lactation		
under 18 y	19 (28.9 IU)	800 (120 IU)
19–50 y	19 (28.9 IU)	1,000 (150 IU)

RDA = Recommended Dietary Allowances
*AI = Adequate Intake
UL = Tolerable Upper Intake Value
ND = not determined
mg = milligram; d = day
1 IU of vitamin E equals 0.66 mg of d- and 0.45 mg of
dl-alpha-tocopherol

The values are adapted and summarized from the tables of the Dietary Reference Intakes (DRI)
published by www.nap.edu.

TABLE A.4. DIETARY REFERENCE
INTAKES (DRI) OF VITAMIN D

Age	RDA/AI*	UL
	µg/d (IU/d)	µg/d (IU/d)
Infants		
0–12 mo	5 (200 IU)*	25 (1,000 IU)
Children		
1–8 y	5 (200 IU)*	50 (2,000 IU)
Males		
9–50 y	5 (200 IU)*	50 (2,000 IU)
50–70 y	10 (400 IU)*	50 (2,000 IU)
over 70 y	15 (600 IU)*	50 (2,000 IU)
Females		
9–50 y	5 (200 IU)*	50 (2,000 IU)
50–70 y	10 (400 IU)*	50 (2,000 IU)
under 70 y	15 (600 IU)*	50 (2,000 IU)
Pregnancy		
18–50 y	5 (200 IU)*	50 (2,000 IU)
Lactation		
18–50 y	5 (200 IU)*	50 (2,000 IU)

RDA = Recommended Dietary Allowances
*AI = Adequate Intake
UL = Tolerable Upper Intake Value
µg = microgram; d = day
1 µg of cholecalciferol equals 40 IU (international unit)
of Vitamin D.

The values are adapted and summarized from the tables of the Dietary Reference Intakes (DRI) published by www.nap.edu.

TABLE A.5. DIETARY REFERENCE
INTAKES (DRI) OF VITAMIN B₁ (THIAMINE)

Age	RDA/AI*	UL
	mg/d	mg/d
Infants		
0–6 mo	0.2*	ND
7–12 mo	0.3*	ND
Children		
1–3 y	0.5	ND
4–8 y	0.6	ND
Males		
9–13 y	0.9	ND
14 y and up	1.2	ND
Females		
9–13 y	0.9	ND
14–18 y	1.0	ND
19 y and up	1.1	ND
Pregnancy		
18–50 y	1.4	ND
Lactation		
18–50 y	1.4	ND

RDA = Recommended Dietary Allowances
*AI = Adequate Intake
UL = Tolerable Upper Intake Value
ND = not determined
mg = milligram; d = day

The values are adapted and summarized from the tables of the Dietary Reference Intakes (DRI) published by www.nap.edu.

TABLE A.6. DIETARY REFERENCE
INTAKES (DRI) OF VITAMIN B$_2$ (RIBOFLAVIN)

Age	RDA/AI*	UL
	mg/d	mg/d
Infants		
0–6 mo	0.3*	ND
7–12 mo	0.4*	ND
Children		
1–3 y	0.5	ND
4–8 y	0.6	ND
Males		
9–13 y	0.9	ND
14 y and up	13	ND
Females		
9–13	0.9	ND
14–18 y	1.0	ND
19 y and up	1.1	ND
Pregnancy		
18–50 y	1.4	ND
Lactation		
18–50 y	1.6	ND

RDA = Recommended Dietary Allowances
*AI = Adequate Intake
UL = Tolerable Upper Intake Value
ND = not determined
mg = milligram; d = day

The values are adapted and summarized from the table of the Dietary Reference Intakes (DRI) published by www.nap.edu.

TABLE A.7. DIETARY REFERENCE
INTAKES (DRI) OF VITAMIN B₆

Age	RDA/AI*	UL
	mg/d	mg/d
Infants		
0–6 mo	0.1*	ND
7–12 mo	0.3*	ND
Children		
1–3 y	0.5	30
4–8 y	0.6	40
Males		
9–13 y	1.0	60
14–50 y	1.3	80
50–70 y and up	1.7	100
Females		
9–13 y	1.0	60
14–18 y	1.2	80
19–30 y	1.3	100
50 y and up	1.5	100
Pregnancy		
under 18 y	1.9	80
19–50 y	1.9	100
Lactation		
under 18 y	2.0	80
19–50 y	2.0	100

RDA = Recommended Dietary Allowances
*AI = Adequate Intake
UL = Tolerable Upper Intake Value
ND = not determined
mg = milligram; d = day

The values are adapted and summarized from the table of the Dietary Reference Intakes (DRI) published by www.nap.edu.

TABLE A.8. DIETARY REFERENCE
INTAKES (DRI) OF VITAMIN B_{12} (COBALAMIN)

Age	RDA/AI*	UL
	µg/d	µg/d
Infants		
0–6 mo	0.4*	ND
7–12 mo	0.5*	ND
Children		
1–3 y	0.9	ND
4–8 y	1.2	ND
Males		
9–13 y	1.08	ND
14 y and up	2.4	ND
Females		
9–13 y	1.8	ND
14 y and up	2.4	ND
Pregnancy		
18–50 y	2.6	ND
Lactation		
18–50 y	2.8	ND

RDA = Recommended Dietary Allowances
*AI = Adequate Intake
UL = Tolerable Upper Intake Value
ND = not determined
µg = microgram; d = day

The values are adapted and summarized from the table of the Dietary Reference Intakes (DRI) published by www.nap.edu.

TABLE A.9. DIETARY REFERENCE
INTAKES (DRI) OF VITAMIN PANTOTHENIC ACID

Age	RDA/AI*	UL
	mg/d	mg/d
Infants		
0–6 mo	1.7*	ND
7–12 mo	1.8*	ND
Children		
1–3 y	2*	ND
4–8 y	2*	ND
Males		
9–13 y	4*	ND
14 y and up	5*	ND
Females		
9–13 y	4*	ND
14 y and up	5*	ND
Pregnancy		
18–50 y	6*	ND
Lactation		
18–50 y	7*	ND

RDA = Recommended Dietary Allowances
*AI = Adequate Intake
UL = Tolerable Upper Intake Value
ND = not determined
mg = milligram; d = day

The values are adapted and summarized from the table of the Dietary Reference Intakes (DRI) published by www.nap.edu.

TABLE A.10. DIETARY REFERENCE
INTAKES (DRI) OF VITAMIN NIACIN

Age	RDA/AI*	UL
	mg/d	mg/d
Infants		
0–6 mo	2*	ND
7–12 mo	0.4*	ND
Children		
1–3 y	6.0	10
4–8 y	8.0	15
Males		
9–13 y	12	20
14–50 y	16	30
50 y and up	16	35
Females		
9–13 y	12	20
14–18 y	14	30
19 y and up	14	35
Pregnancy		
under 18 y	18	30
19–50 y	18	35
Lactation		
under 18 y	17	30
19–50 y	17	35

RDA = Recommended Dietary Allowances
*AI = Adequate Intake
UL = Tolerable Upper Intake Value
ND = not determined
mg = milligram; d = day

The values are adapted and summarized from the table of the Dietary Reference Intakes (DRI) published by www.nap.edu

TABLE A.11. DIETARY REFERENCE INTAKES (DRI) OF VITAMIN FOLATE

Age	RDA/AI*	UL
	µg/d	µg/d
Infants		
0–6 mo	65*	ND
7–12 mo	80*	ND
Children		
1–3 y	150	300
4–8 y	200	400
Males		
9–13 y	300	600
14–18 y	400	800
19 y and up	400	1,000
Females		
9–13 y	300	600
14–18 y	400	800
19 y and up	400	1,000
Pregnancy		
under 18 y	600	800
19–50 y	600	1,000
Lactation		
under 18 y	500	800
19–50 y	500	1,000

RDA = Recommended Dietary Allowances
*AI = Adequate Intake
UL = Tolerable Upper Intake Value
ND = not determined
µg = microgram; d = day

The values are adapted and summarized from the table of the Dietary Reference Intakes (DRI) published by www.nap.edu.

TABLE A.12. DIETARY REFERENCE
INTAKES (DRI) OF MICRONUTRIENT BIOTIN

Age	RDA/AI*	UL
	µg/d	µg/d
Infants		
0–6 mo	0.5*	ND
7–12 mo	0.6*	ND
Children		
1–3 y	8*	ND
4–8 y	12*	ND
Males		
9–13 y	20	ND
14–18 y	25	ND
19 y and up	30	ND
Females		
9–13 y	20	ND
14–18 y	25	ND
19 y and up	30	ND
Pregnancy		
under 18 y	30*	ND
19–50 y	30*	ND
Lactation		
under 18 y	35*	ND
19–50 y	35*	ND

RDA = Recommended Dietary Allowances
*AI = Adequate Intake
UL = Tolerable Upper Intake Value
ND = not determined
µg = microgram; d = day

The values are adapted and summarized from the table of the Dietary Reference Intakes (DRI) published by www.nap.edu.

TABLE A.13. DIETARY REFERENCE
INTAKES (DRI) OF MINERAL CALCIUM

Age	RDA/AI*	UL
	mg/d	mg/d
Infants		
0–6 mo	210*	ND
7–12 mo	270*	ND
Children		
1–3 y	500*	2,500
4–8 y	800*	2,500
Males		
9–18 y	1,300*	2,500
19–50 y	1,000*	2,500
51 y and up	1,200*	2,500
Females		
9–8 y	1,300*	2,500
19–50 y	1,000*	2,500
51 y and up	1,200*	2,500
Pregnancy		
under 18 y	1,300*	2,500
19–50 y	1,000*	2,500
Lactation		
under 18 y	1,300*	2,500
19–50 y	1,000*	2,500

RDA = Recommended Dietary Allowances
*AI = Adequate Intake
UL = Tolerable Upper Intake Value
ND = not determined
mg = milligram; d = day

The values are adapted and summarized from the table of the Dietary Reference Intakes (DRI) published by www.nap.edu.

TABLE A.14. DIETARY REFERENCE
INTAKES (DRI) OF MINERAL MAGNESIUM

Age	RDA/AI*	UL
	mg/d	mg/d
Infants		
0–6 mo	30*	ND
7–12 mo	75*	ND
Children		
1–3 y	80	65
4–8 y	130	110
Males		
9–13 y	240	350
14–18 y	410	350
19–30 y	400	350
31 y and up	420	350
Females		
9–13 y	240	350
14–18 y	360	350
31 y and up	320	350
Pregnancy		
under 18 y	400	350
19–30 y	350	350
31–50 y	360	350
Lactation		
under 18 y	360	350
31–50 y	320	350

RDA = Recommended Dietary Allowances
*AI = Adequate Intake
UL = Tolerable Upper Intake Value
ND = not determined
mg = milligram; d = day

The values are adapted and summarized from the table of the Dietary Reference Intakes (DRI) published by www.nap.edu.

TABLE A.15. DIETARY REFERENCE
INTAKES (DRI) OF MINERAL MANGANESE

Age	RDA/AI*	UL
	mg/d	mg/d
Infants		
0–6 mo	0.003*	ND
7–12 mo	0.6*	ND
Children		
1–3 y	1.2 *	2
4–8 y	1.5*	3
Males		
9–13 y	1.9*	6
14–18 y	2.2*	9
19 y and up	2.3*	11
Females		
9–13 y	1.6*	6
14–18 y	1.6 *	9
19 y and up	1.8*	11
Pregnancy		
under 18 y	2.0*	9
19–50 y	2.0*	11
Lactation		
under 18 y	2.6*	9
19–50 y	2.6*	11

RDA = Recommended Dietary Allowances
*AI = Adequate Intake
UL = Tolerable Upper Intake Value
ND = not determined
mg = milligram; d = day

The values are adapted and summarized from the table of the Dietary Reference Intakes (DRI) published by www.nap.edu.

TABLE A.16. DIETARY REFERENCE
INTAKES (DRI) OF MINERAL CHROMIUM

Age	RDA/AI*	UL
	µg/d	µg/d
Infants		
0–6 mo	0.2*	ND
7–12 mo	5.5*	ND
Children		
1–3 y	11*	ND
4–8 y	15*	ND
Males		
9–13 y	25*	ND
14–50 y	35*	ND
51 y and up	30*	ND
Females		
9–13 y	21*	ND
14–18 y	24*	ND
19–50 y	25*	ND
Pregnancy		
under 18 y	29*	ND
19–50 y	30*	ND
Lactation		
under 18 y	44*	ND
19–50 y	45*	ND

RDA = Recommended Dietary Allowances
*AI = Adequate Intake
UL = Tolerable Upper Intake Value
ND = not determined
µg = microgram; d = day

The values are adapted and summarized from the table of the Dietary Reference Intakes (DRI) published by www.nap.edu.

TABLE A.17. DIETARY REFERENCE
INTAKES (DRI) OF MINERAL COPPER

Age	RDA/AI*	UL
	µg/d	µg/d
Infants		
0–6 mo	200*	ND
7–12 mo	220*	ND
Children		
1–3 y	340	1,000
4–8 y	440	3,000
Males		
9–13 y	700	5,000
14–18 y	890	8,000
19 y and up	900	10,000
Females		
9–13 y	700	5,000
14–18 y	890	8,000
19 y and up	900	10,000
Pregnancy		
under 18 y	1,000	8,000
19–50 y	1,000	10,000
Lactation		
under 18 y	1,300	8,000
19–50 y	1,300	10,000

RDA = Recommended Dietary Allowances
*AI = Adequate Intake
UL = Tolerable Upper Intake Value
ND = not determined
µg = microgram; d = day

The values are adapted and summarized from the table of the Dietary Reference Intakes (DRI) published by www.nap.edu.

TABLE A.18. DIETARY REFERENCE
INTAKES (DRI) OF MINERAL IRON

Age	RDA/AI*	UL
	mg/d	mg/d
Infants		
0–6 mo	0.27*	40
7–12 mo	11	40
Children		
1–3 y	7	40
4–8 y	10	40
Males		
9–13 y	8	40
14–18 y	11	45
19 y and up	8	45
Females		
9–13 y	8	40
14–18 y	15	45
19–50 y	18	45
50 y and up	8	45
Pregnancy		
18–50 y	27	45
Lactation		
under 18 y	10	45
19–50 y	9	45

RDA = Recommended Dietary Allowances
*AI = Adequate Intake
UL = Tolerable Upper Intake Value
ND = not determined
mg = milligram; d = day

The values are adapted and summarized from the table of the Dietary Reference Intakes (DRI) published by www.nap.edu.

TABLE A.19. DIETARY REFERENCE
INTAKES (DRI) OF MINERAL SELENIUM

Age	RDA/AI*	UL
	µg/d	µg/d
Infants		
0–6 mo	15*	45
7–12 mo	20*	60
Children		
1–3 y	20	90
4–8 y	30	150
Males		
9–13 y	40	280
14 y and up	55	400
Females		
9–13 y	40	280
14 y and up	55	400
Pregnancy		
18–50 y	60	400
Lactation		
18–50 y	70	400

RDA = Recommended Dietary Allowances
*AI = Adequate Intake
UL = Tolerable Upper Intake Value
ND = not determined
µg = microgram; d = day

The values are adapted and summarized from the table of the Dietary Reference Intakes (DRI) published by www.nap.edu.

TABLE A.20. DIETARY REFERENCE
INTAKES (DRI) OF MINERAL PHOSPHORUS

Age	RDA/AI*	UL
	mg/d	mg/d
Infants		
0–6 mo	100*	ND
7–12 mo	275*	ND
Children		
1–3 y	460	3,000
4–8 y	500	3,000
Males		
9–18 y	1,250	4,000
19–70 y	700	4,000
70 y and up	700	3,000
Females		
9–18 y	1,250	4,000
19–70 y	700	4,000
70 y and up	700	3,000
Pregnancy		
under 18 y	1,250	3,500
19–50 y	700	3,500
Lactation		
under 18 y	1,250	4,000
19–50 y	700	4,000

RDA = Recommended Dietary Allowances
*AI = Adequate Intake
UL = Tolerable Upper Intake Value
ND = not determined
mg = milligram; d = day

The values are adapted and summarized from the table of the Dietary Reference Intakes (DRI) published by www.nap.edu.

TABLE A.21. DIETARY REFERENCE
INTAKES (DRI) OF MINERAL ZINC

Age	RDA/AI*	UL
	mg/d	mg/d
Infants		
0–6	2*	4
7–12 mo	3	5
Children		
1–3 y	3	7
4–8 y	5	12
Males		
9–13 y	8	23
14–18 y	11	34
19 y and up	11	40
Females		
9–13 y	8	23
14–18 y	9	34
19 y and up	8	40
Pregnancy		
under 18 y	12	34
19–50 y	11	40
Lactation		
under 18 y	13	34
19–50 y	12	40

RDA = Recommended Dietary Allowances
*AI = Adequate Intake
UL = Tolerable Upper Intake Value
ND = not determined
mg = milligram; d = day

The values are adapted and summarized from the table of the Dietary Reference Intakes (DRI) published by www.nap.edu.

TABLE A.22. CALORIE CONTENT
OF SELECTED FOODS

Food	Portion size	Calories
Apple	1	80
Banana	1	100
Beans, green cooked	½ cup	18
Bread, whole wheat	1 slice	56
Butter	1 tablespoon	100
Carrot	1 medium	34
Cheese	1 ounce	107–114
Corn on the cob	5½ inches	160
Egg	1 large	80
Ice cream	½ cup	135
Kidney beans, cooked	½ cup	110
Meat	3 ounces	200–250
Milk, whole	1 cup	150
Milk, skim	1 cup	85
Orange	1	65
Peach	1	38
Peanuts	1 ounce	172
Pear	1	100
Peas	½ cup	86
Potato chips	10 chips	115
Rice, cooked	½ cup	110
Shrimp	3 ounces	78
Tuna	3 ounces	78
Yogurt, low fat	1 cup	140

From K. N. Prasad and K. C. Prasad, *Fight Cancer with Vitamins and Supplements: A Guide to Prevention and Treatment*, Rochester, Vt.: Healing Arts Press, 2001.

TABLE A.23. FAT CONTENT
OF SELECTED FOODS

Food	Portion size	Grams/Portion
Avocado	¹/₈	4
Bacon, crisp	2 slices	6
Beef, roast	3 ounces	26
Biscuit	1	4
Bread, whole wheat	1 slice	1
Cheese, cheddar	1 ounce	9
Chicken, baked, with skin	3 ounces	11
Chicken, baked, without skin	3 ounces	6
Cornbread	1 piece	7
Egg, boiled	1	6
Ice cream	½ cup	7
Margarine	1 teaspoon	4
Mayonnaise	1 tablespoon	11
Milk, whole	1 cup	8
Milk, skim	1 cup	1
Oatmeal, cooked	½ cup	1
Peanut butter	1 tablespoon	7
Pork chop	3 ounces	19
Shrimp	3 ounces	0.9
Sour cream	1 tablespoon	3
Tuna	3 ounces	0.9
Vegetable oil	1 teaspoon	5
Yogurt, low fat	1 cup	4

From K. N. Prasad and K. C. Prasad, *Fight Cancer with Vitamins and Supplements: A Guide to Prevention and Treatment*, Rochester, Vt.: Healing Arts Press, 2001.

TABLE A.24. FIBER CONTENT
OF SELECTED FOODS

Food	Portion size	Grams/Portion
Apple, with skin	1	3
Bread, white	1 slice	0.8
Bread, whole wheat	1 slice	1.3
Broccoli	½ cup	3.2
Carrot, raw	1 medium	2.4
Cereal, all-bran	1 cup	25.6
Cereal, raisin bran	1 cup	6
Corn	½ cup	4.6
Muffin, bran	1	4.2
Pear, with skin	1	3.8
Raspberries	½ cup	4.6

From K. N. Prasad and K. C. Prasad, *Fight Cancer with Vitamins and Supplements: A Guide to Prevention and Treatment*, Rochester, Vt.: Healing Arts Press, 2001.

Abbreviations and Terminologies

AA: Arachidonic acid is a 20-carbon fatty acid that is derived from dietary sources or is formed from linoleic acid, an essential fatty acid

ALA: Alpha-linolenic acid, omega-3 fatty acid derived from plants

Angina: Chest pain, a symptom of heart disease

Antioxidant: An antioxidant is a substance, either a nutrient or an enzyme, which counters the effects of oxidation in the body

CAD: Coronary artery disease

Cardiomyopathy: Damage to heart muscle cells, which impairs the heart's ability to function normally over time

Carotid IMT: Intima medial thickness of a carotid artery or the thickness of the wall of the carotid artery

CHD: Coronary heart disease

CRP: C-reactive protein is one of the protein markers of inflammation present in the blood; it is elevated in heart disease

CVD: Cardiovascular disease

DHA: Docosahexaenoic acid, a form of omega-3 fatty acid derived from fish

Diastole: Contraction of the heart is referred to as *systole* and relaxation of the heart is referred to as *diastole*. During the diastolic process, as the ventricles of the heart relax, they fill the left atrium and the right atrium with blood

DRI: Daily Recommended Intakes

Endothelial dysfunction: Abnormal function of the blood vessels, which typically precedes the development of atherosclerosis

EPA: Eicosapentaenoic acid, a form of omega-3 fatty acid derived from fish

FMD: Flow-mediated dilation, an endothelial-dependent flow-mediated dilation of a blood vessel, which measures its function

Free Iron: Free iron in the blood is iron that is not bound to any proteins; it is a source of oxidative stress

Half-life: The time necessary to remove a substance from the blood by half

HDL cholesterol: High density lipoprotein-cholesterol, higher levels of which are useful in preventing heart disease

Hp: Haptoglobin is an antioxidant protein that protects against oxidative damage

Hypertension: High blood pressure

IL-6: Interleukin-6, a pro-inflammatory cytokine

IMT: Intima media thickness, also defined as the thickness of the wall of a blood vessel. Increased IMT of the carotid artery is often associated with an increased risk of heart disease and stroke due to narrowing of the artery

Incidence: Annual rate of disease occurrence

Ischemia: A condition wherein the heart does not receive enough oxygen due to a poor blood supply to the heart

LDL cholesterol: Low-density lipoprotein cholesterol is the oxidized form of LDL cholesterol; elevated levels of it increase one's risk of developing heart disease

MDA: Malondialdehyde, a marker of oxidative stress and an organic compound that is one of the most frequently used indicators of lipid peroxidation

MI: Myocardial infarction, also called heart attack

NAC: N-acetylcysteine, a common exogenous synthetic antioxidant

NAD+: Nicotinamide adenine dinucleotide, an oxidizing agent

NADH: The reduced form of NAD+, a reducing agent

Nitrosylative damage: Damage produced by free radicals derived from nitrogen

NMD: Nitroglycerine-mediated dilation, an endothelial-independent nitroglycerine-mediated dilation of a blood vessel, which measures its function

NO: Nitric oxide is a substance produced by the body that aids in dilation of blood vessels

NOS: Nitric oxide synthase, an enzyme that makes NO

Oxidation: A process in which an atom or molecule gains oxygen, loses hydrogen, or loses an electron

Oxidative damage: Damage produced by free radicals derived from oxygen

Oxidative stress: When the production of free radicals surpasses the antioxidant capacity of the body to neutralize them

Oxidized LDL cholesterol: LDL cholesterol that has been damaged by free radicals

Prevalence: The total number of people with a disease in a population at a given time

Prooxidant: A substance that hastens the oxidation of another substance either by inhibiting an antioxidant system or through the generation of reactive oxygen species (ROS)

RDA: Recommended Dietary Allowances

Reduction: A process in which an atom or molecule loses oxygen, gains hydrogen, or gains an electron

ROS: Reactive oxygen species are free radicals derived from oxygen

SOD: Superoxide dismutase, an antioxidant enzyme made in the body

Systole: Relaxation of the heart is referred to as *diastole* and contraction of the heart is referred to as *systole*. During the systolic process, as the ventricles of the heart contract, they squeeze blood into blood vessels leading to the lungs

TNF-alpha: Tumor necrosis factor-alpha, a pro-inflammatory cytokine

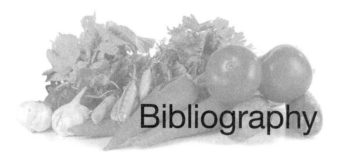

Bibliography

Abate, A., G. Yang, P. A. Dennery, et al. 2000. Synergistic inhibition of cyclooxygenase-2 expression by vitamin E and aspirin. *Free Radical Biology and Medicine* 29, no. 11:1135–42.

Aukrust, P., L. Gullestad, K. T. Lappegard, et al. 2001. Complement activation in patients with congestive heart failure: effect of high-dose intravenous immunoglobulin treatment. *Circulation* 104, no. 13: 1494–1500.

Basili, S., G. Tanzilli, E. Mangieri, et al. 2010. Intravenous ascorbic acid infusion improves myocardial perfusion grade during elective percutaneous coronary intervention: relationship with oxidative stress markers. *JACC: Cardiovascular Interventions* 3, no. 2: 221–29.

Becker, A. E., O. J. de Boer, and A. C. van Der Wal. 2001. The role of inflammation and infection in coronary artery disease. *Annual Review of Medicine* 52: 289–97.

Behrendt, D., J. Beltrame, H. Hikiti, et al. 2006. Impact of coronary endothelial function on the progression of cardiac transplant-associated arteriosclerosis: effect of anti-oxidant vitamins C and E. *Journal of Heart Lung Transplant* 25, no. 4: 426–33.

Belardinelli, R., A. Mucaj, F. Lacalaprice, et al. 2006. Coenzyme Q10 and exercise training in chronic heart failure. *European Heart Journal* 27, no. 22: 2675–81.

Bendinelli, B., G. Masala, C. Saieva, et al. 2011. Fruit, vegetables, and olive oil and risk of coronary heart disease in Italian women: the EPICOR Study. *American Journal of Clinical Nutrition* 93, no. 2: 275–83.

Bergamini, C., M. Cicoira, A. Rossi, et al. 2009. Oxidative stress and hyperuricaemia: pathophysiology, clinical relevance, and therapeutic implications in chronic heart failure. *European Journal of Heart Failure* 11, no. 5: 444–52.

Bertelli, A. A. and D. K. Das. 2009. Grapes, wines, resveratrol and heart health. *Journal of Cardiovascular Pharmacology* 54: 468–76.

Bohm, V. 2012. Lycopene and heart health. *Molecular nutrition & food research* 56, no. 2: 296–303.

Bonaa, K. H., I. Njolstad, P. M. Ueland, et al. 2006. Homocysteine lowering and cardiovascular events after acute myocardial infarction. *New Engand Journal of Medicine* 354, no. 15: 1578–88.

Boone, J. L., and K. N. Prasad. 2009. "Multivitamin Antioxidant Micronutrient Reversal of Intima-Medial Thickness of the Carotid Artery (The MAVRIC Trial)." BraveHeart Program. Denver, Colo.: Boone Heart Institute.

Brouwer, I. A., M. H. Raitt, C. Dullemeijer, et al. 2009. Effect of fish oil on ventricular tachyarrhythmia in three studies in patients with implantable cardioverter defibrillators. *European Heart Journal* 30, no. 7: 820–26.

Brown, B. G., X. Q. Zhao, A. Chait, 2001. Simvastatin and niacin, antioxidant vitamins, or the combination for the prevention of coronary disease. *New England Journal of Medicine* 345, no. 22: 1583–92.

Calo, L., L. Bianconi, F. Colivicchi, et al. 2005. N-3 fatty acids for the prevention of atrial fibrillation after coronary artery bypass surgery: a randomized, controlled trial. *Journal of American College of Cardiology* 45, no. 10: 1723–28.

Canton, M., S. Menazza, F. L. Sheeran, et al. 2011. Oxidation of myofibrillar proteins in human heart failure. *Journal of American College of Cardiology* 57, no. 3: 300–309.

CDC Report. 2010. "Prevalence of Coronary Heart Disease 2006–2010." www.cdc.gov/mmwr/preview/mmwrhtml/mm6040a1.htm. Accessed July 23, 2014.

Chae, C. U., C. M. Albert, M. V. Moorthy, et al. 2012. Vitamin E supplementation and the risk of heart failure in women. *Circulation: Heart Failure* 5, no. 2: 176–82.

Chen, J. W., Y. H. Chen, and S. J. Lin. 2006. Long-term exposure to oxidized low-density lipoprotein enhances tumor necrosis factor-alpha-stimulated endothelial adhesiveness of monocytes by activating superoxide generation and redox-sensitive pathways. *Free Radicals Biology and Medicine* 40, no. 5: 817–26.

Chen, Y. R., F. F. Yi, X. Y. Li, et al. 2008. Resveratrol attenuates ventricular arrhythmias and improves the long-term survival in rats with myocardial infarction. *Cardiovascular Drugs Therapy* 22, no. 6: 479–85.

Cheung, M. C., X. Q. Zhao, A. Chait, et al. 2001. Antioxidant supplements block the response of HDL to simvastatin-niacin therapy in patients with coronary artery disease and low HDL. *Arteriosclerosis, Thrombosis, and Vascular Biology* 21, no. 8: 1320–26.

Choi, B. C. 2000. A technique to re-assess epidemiologic evidence in light of the healthy worker effect: the case of firefighting and heart disease. *Journal of Occupational Environmental Medicine* 42, no. 10: 1021–34.

Cicero, A. F., S. Ertek, and C. Borghi. 2009. Omega-3 polyunsaturated fatty acids: their potential role in blood pressure prevention and management. *Current Vascular Pharmacology* 7, no. 3: 330–37.

Collins, R., R. Peto, and J. Armitage. 2002. The MRC/BHF heart protection study: preliminary results. *International Journal of Clinical Practice* 56, no. 1: 53–56.

Cotran, R. S., V. Kumar, and T. Collins, ed. *Robbins Pathological Basis of Disease,* 6th ed. New York: WB Saunders Company. 543–99.

Cotter, G., E. Shemesh, M. Zehavi, et al. 2004. Lack of aspirin effect: aspirin resistance or resistance to taking aspirin? *American Heart Journal* 147, no. 2: 293–300.

Dagenais, G. R., Q. Yi, E. Lonn, et al. 2005. Impact of cigarette smoking in high-risk patients participating in a clinical trial. A substudy from the Heart Outcomes Prevention Evaluation (HOPE) trial. *European Journal of Cardiovascular Prevention and Rehabilitation* 12, no. 1: 75–81.

Dai, D. F., and P. S. Rabinovitch. 2009. Cardiac aging in mice and humans: the role of mitochondrial oxidative stress. *Trends in Cardiovascular Medicine* 19, no. 7: 213–20.

Dai, Y. L., T. H. Luk, K. H. Yiu, et al. 2011. Reversal of mitochondrial dysfunction by coenzyme Q10 supplement improves endothelial function in patients with ischaemic left ventricular systolic dysfunction: a randomized controlled trial. *Atherosclerosis* 216, no. 2: 395–401.

Danesh, J., and M. B. Pepys. 2009. C-reactive protein and coronary disease: is there a causal link? *Circulation* 120, no. 21: 2036–39.

Danesh, J., J. G. Wheeler, G. M. Hirschfield, et al. 2004. C-reactive protein and other circulating markers of inflammation in the prediction of coronary heart disease. *New England Journal of Medicine* 350, no. 14: 1387–97.

Davies, K. J., and R. Shringarpure. 2006. Preferential degradation of oxidized proteins by the 20S proteasome may be inhibited in aging and in inflammatory neuromuscular diseases. *Neurology* 66, no. 2(1): S93–96.

de Nigris, F., T. Youssef, S. Ciafre, et al. 2000. Evidence for oxidative activation of c-Myc-dependent nuclear signaling in human coronary smooth muscle cells and in early lesions of Watanabe heritable hyperlipidemic rabbits: protective effects of vitamin E. *Circulation* 102, no. 17: 2111–17.

DeMaio, S. J., S. B. King, N. J. Lembo, et al. 1992. Vitamin E supplementation, plasma lipids and incidence of restenosis after percutaneous transluminal coronary angioplasty (PTCA). *Journal of American College of Nutrition* 11, no. 1: 68–73.

Devaraj, S., and I. Jialal. 2000. Alpha-tocopherol supplementation decreases serum C-reactive protein and monocyte interleukin-6 levels in normal volunteers and type 2 diabetic patients. *Free Radicals Biology and Medicine* 29, no. 8: 790–92.

Devaraj, S., R. Tang, B. Adams-Huet, et al. 2007. Effect of high-dose alpha-tocopherol supplementation on biomarkers of oxidative stress and inflammation and carotid atherosclerosis in patients with coronary artery disease. *American Journal of Clinical Nu*trition 86, no. 5: 1392–98.

Devika, P. T., and P. Stanely Mainzen Prince. 2008. (-)Epigallocatechin-gallate (EGCG) prevents mitochondrial damage in isoproterenol-induced cardiac toxicity in albino Wistar rats: a transmission electron microscopic and in vitro study. *Pharmacological Research* 57, no. 5: 351–57.

Dietrich, T., R. I. Garcia, P. de Pablo, et al. 2007. The effects of cigarette smoking on C-reactive protein concentrations in men and women and its modification by exogenous oral hormones in women. *European Journal of Cardiovascular Prevention Rehabilitation* 14, no. 5: 694–700.

Dimitrow, P. P., and M. Jawien. 2009. Pleiotropic, cardioprotective effects of omega-3 polyunsaturated fatty acids. *Mini Review in Medicinal Chemistry* 9, no. 9: 1030–39.

Drexler, H. 1999. Nitric oxide and coronary endothelial dysfunction in humans. *Cardiovascular Research* 43, no. 3: 572–79.

Dudley, J. I., I. Lekli, S. Mukherjee. 2008. Does white wine qualify for French paradox? Comparison of the cardioprotective effects of red and white wines and their constituents: resveratrol, tyrosol, and hydroxytyrosol. *Journal of Agriculture Food and Chemistry* 56, no. 20: 9362–73.

Duthie, G. G., J. R. Arthur, and W. P. James. 1991. Effects of smoking and vitamin E on blood antioxidant status. *American Journal of Clinical Nutrition* 53, 4:1061S–63S.

Earnest, C. P., K. A. Wood, and T. S. Church. 2003. Complex multivitamin supplementation improves homocysteine and resistance to LDL-C oxidation. *Journal of American College of Nutrition* 22, no. 5: 400–407.

El-Hamamsy, I., L. M. Stevens, M. Carrier, et al. 2007. Effect of intravenous n-acetylcysteine on outcomes after coronary artery bypass surgery: a randomized, double-blind, placebo-controlled clinical trial. *Journal of Thoracic Cardiovascular Surgery* 133, no. 1: 7–12.

Fang, J. C., S. Kinlay, J. Beltrame, et al. 2002. Effect of vitamins C and E on progression of transplant-associated arteriosclerosis: a randomised trial. *Lancet* 359 no. 9312: 1108–13.

Folkers, K., P. Langsjoen, and P. H. Langsjoen. 1992. Therapy with coenzyme Q10 of patients in heart failure who are eligible or ineligible for a transplant. *Biochemical and Biophysical Research Communications* 182 no. 1: 247–53.

Freedman, J. E., J. H. Farhat, J. Loscalzo, et al. 1996. Alpha-tocopherol inhibits aggregation of human platelets by a protein kinase C-dependent mechanism. *Circulation* 94, no. 10: 2434–40.

Gey, K. F., and P. Puska. 1989. Plasma vitamins E and A inversely correlated to mortality from ischemic heart disease in cross-cultural epidemiology. *Annals of New York Academy of Sciences* 570: 268–82.

Golias, C., E. Tsoutsi, A. Matziridis, et al. 2007. Review. Leukocyte and endothelial cell adhesion molecules in inflammation focusing on inflammatory heart disease. *In Vivo* 21 no. 5: 757–69.

Grad, E., R. M. Pachino, and H. D. Danenberg. 2011. Endothelial C-reactive protein increases platelet adhesion under flow conditions. *American Journal of Physiology Heart and Circulatory Physiology* 301, no. 3: H730–36.

Gu, W. J., Z. J. Wu, P. F. Wang, et al. 2012. N-Acetylcysteine supplementation for the prevention of atrial fibrillation after cardiac surgery: a meta-analysis of eight randomized controlled trials. *BMC Cardiovascular Disorders* 12: 10.

Gum, P. A., K. Kottke-Marchant, P. A. Welsh, et al. 2003. A prospective, blinded determination of the natural history of aspirin resistance among stable patients with cardiovascular disease. *Journal of the American College of Cardiology* 41, no. 6: 961–65.

Gum, P. A., M. Thamilarasan, J. Watanabe, et al. 2001. Aspirin use and all-cause mortality among patients being evaluated for known or suspected coronary artery disease: a propensity analysis. *Journal of the American Medical Association* 286, no. 10: 1187–94.

Guyton, A. C., and J. E. Hall. 2006. "Cardiac arrhythmias and their electrocardiographic interpretation." *Textbook of Medical Physiology.* 11th ed. New York: Saunders. 136–46.

Harling, L., S. Rasoli, J. A. Vecht, et al. 2011. Do antioxidant vitamins have an anti-arrhythmic effect following cardiac surgery? A meta-analysis of randomised controlled trials. *Heart* 97, no. 20: 1636–42.

He, K. 2009. Fish, long-chain omega-3 polyunsaturated fatty acids and prevention of cardiovascular disease—eat fish or take fish oil supplement? *Progress in Cardiovascular Disease* 52, no. 2: 95–114.

He, L., B. Liu, Z. Dai, et al. 2012. Alpha lipoic acid protects heart against myocardial ischemia-reperfusion injury through a mechanism involving aldehyde dehydrogenase 2 activation. *European Journal of Pharmacology* 678, nos. 1–3: 32–38.

Hecht, H. S., and H. R. Superko. 2001. Electron beam tomography and National Cholesterol Education Program guidelines in asymptomatic women. *Journal of American College of Cardiology* 37, no. 6: 1506–11.

Heidt, M. C., M. Vician, S. K. Stracke, et al. 2009. Beneficial effects of intravenously administered N-3 fatty acids for the prevention of atrial fibrillation after coronary artery bypass surgery: a prospective randomized study. *Thoracic Cardiovasular Surgery* 57, no. 5: 276–80.

Heitzer, T., S. Yla Herttuala, E. Wild, et al. 1999. Effect of vitamin E on endothelial vasodilator function in patients with hypercholesterolemia, chronic smoking or both. *Journal of the American College of Cardiology* 33, no. 2: 499–505.

Hillis, G. S., and A. D. Flapan. 1998. Cell adhesion molecules in cardiovascular disease: a clinical perspective. *Heart* 79, no. 5: 429–31.

Hodis, H. N., W. J. Mack, L. LaBree, et al. 1995. Serial coronary angiographic evidence that antioxidant vitamin intake reduces progression of coronary artery atherosclerosis. *Journal of the American Medical Association* 273, no. 23: 1849–54.

Holub, B. J. 2009. Docosahexaenoic acid (DHA) and cardiovascular disease risk factors. *Prostaglandins, Leukotreines, and Essential Fatty Acids* 81, no. 2–3: 199–204.

Holvoet, P., and D. Collen. 1994. Oxidized lipoproteins in atherosclerosis and thrombosis. *FASEB Journal* 8, no. 15: 1279–84.

Ingold, K. U., G. W. Burton, D. O. Foster, et al. 1987. Biokinetics of and discrimination between dietary RRR- and SRR-alpha-tocopherols in the male rat. *Lipids* 22, no. 3: 163–72.

Islam, K. N., D. O'Byrne, S. Devaraj, et al. 2000. Alpha-tocopherol supplementation decreases the oxidative susceptibility of LDL in renal failure patients on dialysis therapy. *Atherosclerosis* 150, no. 1: 217–24.

Jaxa-Chamiec, T., B. Bednarz, K. Herbaczynska-Cedro, et al. 2009. Effects of vitamins C and E on the outcome after acute myocardial infarction in diabetics: a retrospective, hypothesis-generating analysis from the MIVIT study. *Cardiology* 112, no. 3: 219–23.

Jenkins, D. J., A. R. Josse, P. Dorian, et al. 2008. Heterogeneity in randomized controlled trials of long chain (fish) omega-3 fatty acids in restenosis, secondary prevention and ventricular arrhythmias. *Journal of the American College of Nutrition* 27, no. 3: 367–78.

Joseph, J., L. Joseph, S. Devi, et al. 2008. Effect of anti-oxidant treatment on hyperhomocysteinemia-induced myocardial fibrosis and diastolic dysfunction. *Journal of Heart Lung and Transplant* 27, no. 11: 1237–41.

Judy, W. V., Folkers, K., and J. H. Hall. 1991. Improved long-term survival in coenzyme Q10 treated congestive heart failure patients compared to conventionally treated patients. *Biomedical and Clincial Aspects of Coenzyme Q.* (Amsterdam) 291–98.

Kales, S. N., E. S. Soteriades, C. A. Christophi, et al. 2007. Emergency duties and deaths from heart disease among firefighters in the United States. *New England Journal of Medicine* 356, no. 12: 1207–15.

Karppi, J., S. Kurl, J. A. Laukkanen, et al. 2011. Plasma carotenoids are related to intima media thickness of the carotid artery wall in men from eastern Finland. *Journal of Internal Medicine* 270, no. 5: 478–485.

Karter, Jr., M. J., and J. A. Molis. "Fire fighter injuries—2006." *National Fire Protection Association.* November 2007.

Kelemen, M., D. Vaidya, D. D. Waters, et al. 2005. Hormone therapy and antioxidant vitamins do not improve endothelial vasodilator function in postmenopausal women with established coronary artery disease: a substudy of the Women's Angiographic Vitamin and Estrogen (WAVE) trial. *Atherosclerosis* 179, no. 1: 193–200.

Kennedy, A. R., and N. I Krinsky. 1994. Effects of retinoids, beta-carotene, and canthaxanthin on UV- and X-ray-induced transformation of C3H10T1/2 cells in vitro. *Nutrition and Cancer* 22, no. 3: 219–32.

Kinlay, S., D. Behrendt, J. C. Fang, et al. 2004. Long-term effect of combined vitamins E and C on coronary and peripheral endothelial function. *Journal of the American College of Cardiology* 43, no. 4: 629–34.

Knekt, P., J. Ritz, M. A. Pereira, et al. 2004. Antioxidant vitamins and coronary heart disease risk: a pooled analysis of 9 cohorts. *American Journal of Clinical Nutrition* 80, no. 6: 1508–20.

Koh, W. P., J. M. Yuan, R. Wang, et al. 2011. Plasma carotenoids and risk of acute myocardial infarction in the Singapore Chinese Health Study. *Nutrition, Metabolism, and Cardiovascular Diseases* 21, no. 9: 685–90.

Kromhout, D., J. M. Geleijnse, J. de Goede, 2011. N-3 fatty acids, ventricular arrhythmia-related events, and fatal myocardial infarction in postmyocardial infarction patients with diabetes. *Diabetes Care* 34, no. 12: 2515–20.

Kubota, Y., H. Iso, C. Date, et al. 2011. Dietary intakes of antioxidant vitamins and mortality from cardiovascular disease: the Japan Collaborative Cohort Study (JACC) study. *Stroke* 42, no. 6: 1665–72.

Kumar, A., A. R. Hovland, F. G. La Rosa, et al. 2000. Relative sensitivity of undifferentiated and cyclic adenosine 3',5'-monophosphate-induced differentiated neuroblastoma cells to cyclosporin A: potential role of beta-amyloid and ubiquitin in neurotoxicity. *In Vitro Cellular and Developmental Biology—Animal* 36, no. 2: 81–87.

Langsjoen, P. H., P. H. Langsjoen, and K. Folkers. 1990. Long-term efficacy and safety of coenzyme Q10 therapy for idiopathic dilated cardiomyopathy. *American Journal of Cardiology* 65, no. 7: 521–23.

Lavie, C. J., R. V. Milani, M. R. Mehra, et al. 2009. Omega-3 polyunsaturated fatty acids and cardiovascular diseases. *Journal of the American College of Cardiology* 54, no. 7: 585–94.

Leander, K., J. Hallqvist, C. Reuterwall, et al. 2001. Family history of coronary heart disease, a strong risk factor for myocardial infarction interacting with other cardiovascular risk factors: results from the Stockholm Heart Epidemiology Program (SHEEP). *Epidemiology* 12, no. 2: 215–21.

Lee, B. J., Y. C. Huang, S. J. Chen, et al. 2012a. Coenzyme Q10 supplementation reduces oxidative stress and increases antioxidant enzyme activity in patients with coronary artery disease. *Nutrition* 28, no. 3: 250–55.

Lee, B. J., Y. C. Huang, S. J. Chen, et al. 2012b. Effects of coenzyme Q10 supplementation on inflammatory markers (high-sensitivity C-reactive protein, interleukin-6, and homocysteine) in patients with coronary artery disease. *Nutrition* 28, no. 7–8: 767–72.

Lee, J. H., J. H. O'Keefe, C. J. Lavie, et al. 2009. Omega-3 fatty acids: cardiovascular benefits, sources and sustainability. *Nature Reviews Cardiology*.

Leppala, J. M., J. Virtamo, R. Fogelholm, et al. 2000. Controlled trial of alpha-tocopherol and beta-carotene supplements on stroke incidence and mortality in male smokers. *Arteriosclerosis, Thrombosis, and Vascular Biology* 20, no. 1: 230–35.

Levy, A. P., P. Friedenberg, R. Lotan, et al. 2004. The effect of vitamin therapy on the progression of coronary artery atherosclerosis varies by haptoglobin type in postmenopausal women. *Diabetes Care* 27, no. 4: 925–30.

Li, L., N. Roumeliotis, T. Sawamura, et al. 2004. C-reactive protein enhances LOX-1 expression in human aortic endothelial cells: relevance of LOX-1 to C-reactive protein-induced endothelial dysfunction. *Circulation Research* 95, no. 9: 877–83.

Littarru, G. P., L. Tiano, R. Belardinelli, et al. 2011. Coenzyme Q(10), endothelial function, and cardiovascular disease. *Biofactors* 37, no. 5: 366–73.

Liu, L., and M. Meydani. 2002. Combined vitamin C and E supplementation retards early progression of arteriosclerosis in heart transplant patients. *Nutrition Reviews* 60, no. 11: 368–71.

Lombardi, F., and P. Terranova. 2007. Anti-arrhythmic properties of N-3 polyunsaturated fatty acids (N-3 PUFA). *Current Medicinal Chemistry* 14, no. 19: 2070–80.

Lonn, E., J. Bosch, S. Yusuf, et al. 2005. Effects of long-term vitamin E supplementation on cardiovascular events and cancer: a randomized controlled trial. *Journal of the American Medical Association* 293, no. 11: 1338–47.

Lonn, E., S. Yusuf, M. J. Arnold, et al. 2006. Homocysteine lowering with folic acid and B vitamins in vascular disease. *New England Journal of Medicine* 354, no. 15: 1567–77.

Lonn, E., S. Yusuf, B. Hoogwerf, et al. 2002. Effects of vitamin E on cardiovascular and microvascular outcomes in high-risk patients with diabetes: results of the HOPE study and MICRO-HOPE substudy. *Diabetes Care* 25, no. 11: 1919–27.

Losonczy, K. G., T. B. Harris, and R. J. Havlik. 1996. Vitamin E and vitamin C supplement use and risk of all-cause and coronary heart disease mortality in older persons: the Established Populations for Epidemiologic Studies of the Elderly. *American Journal of Clinical Nutrition* 64 no. 2: 190–96.

Macchi, L., N. Sorel, and L. Christiaens. 2006. Aspirin resistance: definitions, mechanisms, prevalence, and clinical significance. *Current Pharmaceutical Design* 12, no. 2: 251–58.

Malik, T. H., A. Cortini, D. Carassiti, et al. 2010. The alternative pathway is critical for pathogenic complement activation in endotoxin- and diet-induced atherosclerosis in low-density lipoprotein receptor-deficient mice. *Circulation* 122, no. 19: 1948–56.

Mann, J. F., E. M. Lonn, Q. Yi, et al. 2004. Effects of vitamin E on cardiovascular outcomes in people with mild-to-moderate renal insufficiency: results of the HOPE study. *Kidney International* 65, no. 4: 1375–80.

Marchioli, R., G. Levantesi, A. Macchia, et al. 2006. Vitamin E increases the risk of developing heart failure after myocardial infarction: results from GISSI-Prevenzione trial. *Journal of Cardiovascular Medicine* (Hagerstown) 7: 347–50.

Marchioli, R., G. Levantesi, M. G. Silletta, et al. 2009. Effect of N-3 polyunsaturated fatty acids and rosuvastatin in patients with heart failure: results of the GISSI-HF trial. *Expert Review of Cardiovascular Therapy* 7, no. 7: 735–48.

Marchioli, R., M. G. Silletta, G. Levantesi, et al. 2009. Omega-3 fatty acids and heart failure. *Current Atherosclerosis Reports* 11, no. 6: 440–47.

Matthan, N. R., A. Giovanni, E. J. Schaefer, et al. 2003. Impact of simvastatin, niacin, and/or antioxidants on cholesterol metabolism in CAD patients with low HDL. *Journal of Lipid Research* 44, no. 4: 800–806.

Mazzini, M., T. Tadros, D. Siwik, et al. 2011. Primary carnitine deficiency and sudden death: in vivo evidence of myocardial lipid peroxidation and sulfonylation of sarcoendoplasmic reticulum calcium ATPase 2. *Cardiology* 120, no. 1: 52–58.

McKechnie, R., M. Rubenfire, and L. Mosca. 2002. Antioxidant nutrient supplementation and brachial reactivity in patients with coronary artery disease. *Journal of Laboratory and Clinical Medicine* 139, no. 3: 133–39.

McMackin, C. J., M. E. Widlansky, N. M. Hamburg, et al. 2007. Effect of combined treatment with alpha-Lipoic acid and acetyl-L-carnitine on vascular function and blood pressure in patients with coronary artery disease. *Journal of Clinical Hypertension* (Greenwich) 9, no. 4: 249–55.

Mente, A., L. de Koning, H. S. Shannon, et al. 2009. A systematic review of the evidence supporting a causal link between dietary factors and coronary heart disease. *Archives of Internal Medicine* 169, no. 7: 659–69.

Montero, I., J. Orbe, N. Varo, et al. 2006. C-reactive protein induces matrix metalloproteinase-1 and -10 in human endothelial cells: implications for clinical and subclinical atherosclerosis. *Journal of the American College of Cardiology* 47, no. 7: 1369–78.

Moolenaar, R. L., ed. 2010. "Prevalence of Coronary Heart Disease—United States, 2006–2010." *Morbidity and Morality Weekly Report* 60, no. 40.

Mori, T. A., V. Burke, I. Puddey, et al. 2009. The effects of [omega]3 fatty acids and coenzyme Q10 on blood pressure and heart rate in chronic kidney disease: a randomized controlled trial. *Journal of Hypertension* 27, no. 9: 1863–72.

Movahed, A., L. Yu, S. J. Thandapilly, et al. 2012. Resveratrol protects adult cardiomyocytes against oxidative stress mediated cell injury. *Archives of Biochemistry Biophysics* 527: 74–80.

Murr, C., B. M. Winklhofer-Roob, K. Schroecksnadel, et al. 2009. Inverse association between serum concentrations of neopterin and antioxidants in patients with and without angiographic coronary artery disease. *Atherosclerosis* 202, no. 2: 543–49.

Myint, P. K., R. N. Luben, N. J. Wareham, et al. 2011. Association between plasma vitamin C concentrations and blood pressure in the European prospective investigation into cancer-Norfolk population-based study. *Hypertension* 58, no. 3: 372–79.

Neunteufl, T., K. Kostner, R. Katzenschlager, et al. 1998. Additional benefit of vitamin E supplementation to simvastatin therapy on vasoreactivity of the brachial artery of hypercholesterolemic men. *Journal of the American College of Cardiology* 32, no. 3: 711–16.

Niwano, S., H. Niwano, S. Sasaki, et al. 2011. N-acetylcysteine suppresses the progression of ventricular remodeling in acute myocarditis: studies in an experimental autoimmune myocarditis (EAM) model. *Circulation Journal* 75, no. 3: 662–71.

Odden, M. C., P. G. Coxson, A. Moran, et al. 2011. The impact of the aging population on coronary heart disease in the United States. *American Journal of Medicine* 124, no. 9: 827–33.

Onat, A., G. Hergenc, G. Can, et al. 2010. Serum complement C3: a determinant of cardiometabolic risk, additive to the metabolic syndrome, in middle-aged population. *Metabolism: Clinical and Experimental* 59, no. 5: 628–34.

Papoulidis, P., O. Ananiadou, E. Chalvatzoulis, et al. 2011. The role of ascorbic acid in the prevention of atrial fibrillation after elective on-pump myocardial revascularization surgery: a single-center experience—a pilot study. *Interactive Cardiovascular and Thoracic Surgery* 12, no. 2: 121–24.

Pasceri, V., J. S. Cheng, J. T. Willerson, et al. 2001. Modulation of C-reactive protein-mediated monocyte chemoattractant protein-1 induction in human endothelial cells by anti-atherosclerosis drugs. *Circulation* 103, no. 21: 2531–34.

Patel, D., and M. Moonis. 2007. Clinical implications of aspirin resistance. *Expert Review of Cardiovascular Therapy* 5, no. 5: 969–75.

Patterson, A. J., D. Xiao, F. Xiong, et al. 2012. Hypoxia-derived oxidative stress mediates epigenetic repression of PKCepsilon gene in foetal rat hearts. *Cardiovascular Research* 93, no. 2: 302–10.

Penumathsa, S. V., and N. Maulik. 2009. Resveratrol: a promising agent in promoting cardioprotection against coronary heart disease. *Canadian Journal of Physiology and Pharmacology* 87, no. 4: 275–86.

Perez-de-Arce, K., R. Foncea, and F. Leighton. 2005. Reactive oxygen species mediates homocysteine-induced mitochondrial biogenesis in human endothelial cells: modulation by antioxidants. *Biochemical Biophysical Research Communication* 338, no. 2: 1103–109.

Perez-Vizcaino, F., and J. Duarte. 2010. Flavonols and cardiovascular disease. *Molecular Aspects of Medicine* 31, no. 6: 478–94.

Pfister, R., S. J. Sharp, R. Luben, et al. 2011. Plasma vitamin C predicts incident heart failure in men and women in European Prospective Investigation into Cancer and Nutrition—Norfolk prospective study. *American Heart Journal* 162, no. 2: 246–53.

Pignatelli, P., G. Tanzilli, R. Carnevale, et al. 2011. Ascorbic acid infusion blunts CD40L upregulation in patients undergoing coronary stent. *Cardiovascular Therapeutics* 29, no. 6: 385–94.

Plantinga, Y., L. Ghiadoni, A. Magagna, et al. 2007. Supplementation with vitamins C and E improves arterial stiffness and endothelial function in essential hypertensive patients. *American Journal of Hypertension* 20, no. 4: 392–97.

Prasad, K. N. 2011. "Micronutrients in healthy aging." Chap. 4 in *Micronutrients in Health and Disease*. Boca Raton, Fla.: CRC Press.

Prasad, K. N., and K.C. Prasad. 2011. "Free radicals, inflammation, the immune system, and antioxidants." Chap. 3 in *Fighting Cancer with Vitamins and Antioxidants*. Rochester, Vt.: Healing Arts Press. 14–28.

Prasad, K. N., B. Kumar, X. D. Yan, et al. 2003. Alpha-tocopheryl succinate, the most effective form of vitamin E for adjuvant cancer treatment: a review. *Journal of the American College of Nutrition* 22, no. 2: 108–17.

Punithavathi, V. R., and P. Stanely Mainzen Prince. 2011. The cardioprotective effects of a combination of quercetin and alpha-tocopherol on isoproterenol-induced myocardial infarcted rats. *Journal of Biochemical and Molecular Toxicology* 25, no. 1: 28–40.

Qin, F., D. A. Siwik, I. Luptak, et al. 2012. The polyphenols resveratrol and S17834 prevent the structural and functional sequelae of diet-induced metabolic heart disease in mice. *Circulation* 125, no. 14: 1757–64, 1751–56.

Qureshi, A. A., C. W. Karpen, N. Qureshi, et al. 2011. Tocotrienols-induced inhibition of platelet thrombus formation and platelet aggregation in stenosed canine coronary arteries. *Lipids Health and Disease* 10: 58, E-publication ahead of print.

Ray, J. G., C. Kearon, Q. Yi, et al. 2007. Homocysteine-lowering therapy and the risk for venous thromboembolism: a randomized trial. *Anna Interm Med* 146: 761–67.

Reinhart, K. M., C. I. Coleman, C. Teevan, et al. 2008. Effects of garlic on blood pressure in patients with and without systolic hypertension: a meta-analysis. *The Annals of Pharmacotherapy* 42, no. 12: 1766–71.

Reiter, R. J., D. X. Tan, S. D. Paredes, et al. 2010. Beneficial effects of melatonin in cardiovascular disease. *Annals of Medicine* 42, no. 4: 276–85.

Reznick, A. Z., C. E. Cross, M. L Hu, et al. 1992. Modification of plasma proteins by cigarette smoke as measured by protein carbonyl formation. *The Biochemical Journal* 286 (Pt 2): 607–11.

Ridker, P. M., M. Cushman, M. J. Stampfer, et al. 1997. Inflammation, aspirin, and the risk of cardiovascular disease in apparently healthy men. *New England Journal of Medicine* 336, no. 14: 973–79.

Ridker, P. M., C. H. Hennekens, J. E. Buring, et al. 2000. C-reactive protein and other markers of inflammation in the prediction of cardiovascular disease in women. *New England Journal of Medicine* 342, no. 12: 836–43.

Riemersma, R. A., D. A. Wood, C. C. Macintyre, et al. 1991. Risk of angina pectoris and plasma concentrations of vitamins A, C, and E and carotene. *Lancet* 337, no. 8732: 1–5.

Riley, S. J., and G. A. Stouffer. 2002. Cardiology Grand Rounds from the University of North Carolina at Chapel Hill. The antioxidant vitamins and coronary heart disease: Part 1, basic science background and clinical observational studies. *American Journal of Medical Sciences* 324, no. 6: 314–20.

Rimm, E. B., M. J. Stampfer, A. Ascherio, et al. 1993. Vitamin E consumption and the risk of coronary heart disease in men. *New England Journal of Medicine* 328, no. 20: 1450–56.

Sacher, H. L., M. L. Sacher, S. W. Landau, et al. 1997. The clinical and hemodynamic effects of coenzyme Q10 in congestive cardiomyopathy. *American Journal of Therapeutics* 4, nos. 2–3: 66–72.

Salonen, J. T. 2002. Clinical trials testing cardiovascular benefits of antioxidant supplementation. *Free Radical Research* 36, no. 12: 1299–1306.

Schnabel, R. B., M. G. Larson, J. F. Yamamoto, et al. 2009. Relation of multiple inflammatory biomarkers to incident atrial fibrillation. *American Journal of Cardiology* 104, no. 1: 92–96.

Sesso, H. D., W. G. Christen, V. Bubes, et al. 2012. Multivitamins in the prevention of cardiovascular disease in men: the Physicians' Health Study II randomized controlled trial. *Journal of the American Medical Association* 308, no. 17: 1751–60.

Simopoulos, A. P. 2008. The omega-6/omega-3 fatty acid ratio, genetic variation, and cardiovascular disease. *Asia Pacific Journal of Clinical Nutrition* 17, no. 1: 131–34.

Sirker, A., M. Zhang, C. Murdoch, et al. 2007. Involvement of NADPH oxidases in cardiac remodelling and heart failure. *American Journal of Nephrology* 27, no. 6: 649–60.

Sklodowska, R. W., J. Gromadzinska, W. Miroslaw, et al. 1991. Selenium and vitamin E concentrations in plasma and erthrocytes of angina pectoris patients. *Trace Elements in Medicine* 8: 113–17.

Stampfer, M. J., C. H. Hennekens, J. E. Manson, et al. 1993. Vitamin E consumption and the risk of coronary disease in women. *New England Journal of Medicine* 328, no. 20: 1444–49.

Stephens, N. G., A. Parsons, P. M. Schofield, et al. 1996. Randomised controlled trial of vitamin E in patients with coronary disease: Cambridge Heart Antioxidant Study (CHAOS). *Lancet* 347, no. 9004: 781–86.

Sukhanov, S., Y. Higashi, S. Y. Shai, et al. 2007. IGF-1 reduces inflammatory responses, suppresses oxidative stress, and decreases atherosclerosis progression in ApoE-deficient mice. *Arteriosclerosis Thrombosis Vascular Biology* 27, no. 12: 2684–90.

Tanaka, Y., Y. Moritoh, and N. Miwa. 2007. Age-dependent telomere-shortening is repressed by phosphorylated alpha-tocopherol together with cellular longevity and intracellular oxidative-stress reduction in human brain microvascular endotheliocytes. *Journal of Cellular Biochemistry* 102, no. 3: 689–703.

Toole, J. F., M. R. Malinow, L. E. Chambless, et al. 2004. Lowering homocysteine in patients with ischemic stroke to prevent recurrent stroke, myocardial infarction, and death: the Vitamin Intervention for Stroke Prevention (VISP) randomized controlled trial. *Journal of the American Medical Association* 291, no. 5: 565–75.

Tornwall, M. E., J. Virtamo, P. A. Korhonen, et al. 2004a. Postintervention effect of alpha-tocopherol and beta carotene on different strokes: a 6-year follow-up of the Alpha-tocopherol, Beta Carotene Cancer Prevention Study. *Stroke* 35, no. 8: 1908–13.

Tornwall, M. E., J. Virtamo, P. A. Korhonen, et al. 2004b. Effect of alpha-tocopherol and beta-carotene supplementation on coronary heart disease during the 6-year post-trial follow-up in the ATBC study. *European Heart Journal* 25, no. 13: 1171–78.

Tossios, P., W. Bloch, A. Huebner, et al. 2003. N-acetylcysteine prevents reactive oxygen species-mediated myocardial stress in patients undergoing cardiac surgery: results of a randomized, double-blind, placebo-controlled clinical trial. *Journal of Thoracic Cardiovascular Surgery* 126, no. 5: 1513–20.

Troseid, M., I. Seljeflot, E. M. Hjerkinn, et al. 2009. Interleukin-18 is a strong predictor of cardiovascular events in elderly men with the metabolic syndrome: synergistic effect of inflammation and hyperglycemia. *Diabetes Care* 32, no. 3: 486–92.

Tsai, M. S., C. H. Huang, C. Y. Tsai, et al. 2011. Ascorbic acid mitigates the myocardial injury after cardiac arrest and electrical shock. *Intensive Care Medicine* 37, no. 12: 2033–40.

Tsutsui, H., S. Kinugawa, and S. Matsushima. 2011. Oxidative stress and heart failure. *American Journal of Physiology Heart and Circulatory Physiology* 301, no. 6: H2181–90.

USPST Force. 2003. Routine vitamin supplementation to prevent cancer and cardiovascular disease: recommendation and rationale. *Annals of Internal Medicine.* 51–55.

Venugopal, D., M. Zahid, P. C. Mailander, et al. 2008. Reduction of estrogen-induced transformation of mouse mammary epithelial cells by n-acetylcysteine. *The Journal of Steroid Biochemistry and Molecular Biology* 109, no. 1–2: 22–30.

Verlangieri, A. J., and M. J. Bush. 1992. Effects of d-alpha-tocopherol supplementation on experimentally induced primate atherosclerosis. *Journal of the American College of Nutrition* 11, no. 2: 131–38.

Wang, Q., X. Zhu, Q. Xu, et al. 2005. Effect of C-reactive protein on gene expression in vascular endothelial cells. *American Journal of Physiology Heart and Circulatory Physiology* 288, no. 4: H1539–45.

Wang, T. J., H. Parise, D. Levy, et al. 2004. Obesity and the risk of new-onset atrial fibrillation. *Journal of the American Medical Association* 292, no. 20: 2471–77.

Waters, D. D., E. L. Alderman, J. Hsia, et al. 2002. Effects of hormone replacement therapy and antioxidant vitamin supplements on coronary atherosclerosis in postmenopausal women: a randomized controlled trial. *Journal of the American Medical Association* 288, no. 19: 2432–40.

Weinberg, R. B., B. S. VanderWerken, R. A. Anderson, et al. 2001. Pro-oxidant effect of vitamin E in cigarette smokers consuming a high polyunsaturated fat diet. *Arteriosclerosis, Thrombosis, and Vascular Biology* 21, no. 6: 1029–33.

Wright, M. E., K. A. Lawson, S. J. Weinstein, et al. 2006. Higher baseline serum concentrations of vitamin E are associated with lower total and cause-specific mortality in the Alpha-Tocopherol, Beta-Carotene Cancer Prevention Study. *American Journal of Clinical Nutrition* 84, no. 5: 1200–1207.

Wu, J., Y. Wang, Y. Zhang, et al. 2011. Association between interleukin-16 polymorphisms and risk of coronary artery disease. *DNA and Cell Biology* 30, no. 5: 305–308.

Xi, J., H. Wang, R. A. Mueller, et al. 2009. Mechanism for resveratrol-induced cardioprotection against reperfusion injury involves glycogen synthase kinase 3beta and mitochondrial permeability transition pore. *European Journal of Pharmacology* 604, no. 1–3: 111–16.

Xiong, F., D. Xiao, and L. Zhang. 2012. Norepinephrine causes epigenetic repression of PKC [varepsilon] gene in rodent hearts by activating Nox1-dependent reactive oxygen species production. *FASEB Journal* 26: 2753–63.

Yu, W., Y. C. Fu, X. H. Zhou, et al. 2009. Effects of resveratrol on H(2)O(2)-induced apoptosis and expression of SIRTs in H9c2 cells. *Journal of Cell Biochemistry* 107, no. 4: 741–47.

Yusuf, S., G. Dagenais, J. Pogue, et al. 2000. Vitamin E supplementation and cardiovascular events in high-risk patients. The Heart Outcomes Prevention Evaluation Study Investigators. *New England Journal of Medicine* 342, no. 3: 154–60.

Zhang, W., D. Lu, W. Dong, et al. 2011. Expression of CYP2E1 increases oxidative stress and induces apoptosis of cardiomyocytes in transgenic mice. *FEBS Journal* 278, no. 9: 1484–92.

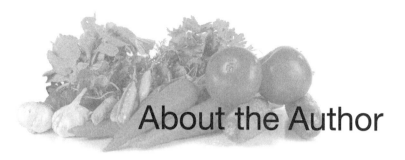

About the Author

Kedar N. Prasad, Ph.D., former president of the International Society for Nutrition and Cancer, obtained a master's degree in zoology from the University of Bihar, Ranchi, India, and his Ph.D. degree in radiation biology from the University of Iowa, Iowa City, in 1963. He then attended the Brookhaven National Laboratory on Long Island for post-doctoral training before joining the Department of Radiology at the University of Colorado Health Sciences Center, where he became a professor in 1980. Later he was appointed director of the Center for Vitamins and Cancer Research at the University of Colorado School of Medicine. In 1982 he was invited by the Nobel Prize Committee to nominate a candidate for the Nobel Prize in medicine, and in 1999 he was selected to deliver the Harold Harper Lecture at the meeting of the American College of Advancement in Medicine.

His published papers and articles have appeared in such illustrious publications as *Science, Nature,* and *Proceedings of the National Academy of Sciences of the United States of America* (PNAS). He is also the author of several book chapters and eighteen books, including *Fighting Cancer with Vitamins and Antioxidants.* A member of several professional organizations, he serves as an ad-hoc member of various study sections of the National Institutes of Health (NIH) and has consistently obtained NIH grants for his research.

Kedar N. Prasad is frequently an invited speaker at national and international meetings on nutrition and cancer. He began researching various types of cancers and the effects of radiation on human tissues in 1963. Over the next twenty-five years, he continued his biological research at five major universities and research labs, studying the relationships between micronutrients, cancer, and radiation and focusing on the effects that micronutrients have on human cells and the manner in which they interact with mainstream medical therapies for many common diseases. He found that certain combinations of micronutrients when taken in conjunction with standard treatments, such as chemotherapy, enhanced and complemented the effects of these traditional therapies. The findings inspired him to further his research to determine the effects that these micronutrient combinations might have on other diseases and on general human health.

His present research interests are in the areas of radiation protection, nutrition and cancer, and nutrition and neurological diseases, particularly Alzheimer's disease and Parkinson's disease. Since 2005 he has been the chief scientific officer of the Premier Micronutrient Corporation, which produces antioxidant micronutrient formulations to fight disease and promote a healthy lifestyle.

Index